Eight Seconds
of MenB

Peter A Smith

Grosvenor House
Publishing Limited

This book is published by
Grosvenor House Publishing Ltd
Link House
140 The Broadway, Tolworth, Surrey, KT6 7HT.
www.grosvenorhousepublishing.co.uk

A CIP record for this book
is available from the British Library

ISBN 978-1-83975-315-2

Thanks to: Philips Electronics UK Limited for their kind
permission to reproduce the background image of the disposable
nebuliser leaflet for the cover.

Contents

Foreword

A few years ago I was invited to give a talk on the laboratory diagnosis of Sepsis which was held at the University of Northampton.

In the audience were a number of people who had had sepsis and survived. I had the opportunity to chat to two of these people, one of which was Peter Smith. He introduced himself as he was curious to get some more detail about some aspects of my talk. The result was a conversation that lasted considerably longer than I anticipated and I was a little late for my next engagement. However I am grateful that my conversation with Peter went on as long as it did. He told me about his encounter with sepsis in quite graphic detail and I was inspired by the courage and fortitude of both men.

Peter took up my invitation to visit the Microbiology Department and I was pleased to be able to show him what the bacteria, *Neisseria meningitidis,* which caused his sepsis looks like under the a light microscope, within the White Blood Cell (count) and how the bacterium is grown and cultivated on agar plates in the laboratory. I was also able to show him how it is tested against a series of antibiotics which could potentially be used as part of the treatment for the disease.

I meet with Peter from time to time where he gave me updates on how he's coping with and manging the sequelae of the sepsis that almost killed him. I gained a lot from my meeting with Pete – inspiration from his miraculous survival, also his fortitude and his determination to enjoy his life with his lovely family.

This one episode teaches us all so much about life.

It is a book of courage and wisdom.

Augustus Lusack,
Northampton General Hospital (NGH)
Head of Pathology, August 2020.

The different text font indicates information taken from my critical care diary that was prepared for me by Nurse Emma Madden.

Text within lines in the other text font are general notes of explanation taken from other sources: The UK Sepsis Trust website, general internet searches, my medical notes and discharge summary.

Chapter One

The confusing beginning

So, I awoke in an unfamiliar room full of medical equipment, surrounded by faces I didn't recognise, not realising that I was already a week into a month that, at best would change my life thereafter or at worst might end it.

Almost a week earlier on the Friday, early in the evening I felt pretty bad with a chill like nothing I'd experienced before, cold to the middle of my bones. A little extra knowledge and a simple £3 digital thermometer would probably have flagged up that this was far from normal. I did what I expect a lot of people might do, I took a Lemsip and went to bed very early, around 8.30pm-ish, thinking I'd got flu and wouldn't be feeling great that weekend.

I had contracted meningococcal bacterial meningitis and would soon develop sepsis and pneumonia, Lemsip Max was not going to be enough.

I would have four and a half weeks in Northampton General Hospital (NGH). Two spells in the Intensive

Care Unit (ICU), amounting to nine days, and three days in the High Dependency Unit (HDU).

I'm not altogether sure when it was that I first became more aware. I think the combination of the bashing my brain was getting from the infection, together with the side effects of the powerful medication that I was on, completely altered my consciousness and perception of everything, I was in a sort of temporary, three-week-long psychosis.

Although this was actually the first time I'd been admitted to hospital. During the second week I concluded that this was at least my third time. On this occasion I'd been forcibly institutionalised around three months earlier, sectioned against my will, in a conspiracy involving my family, the doctors and nurses. I had to stop the unnecessary medication that was subduing me and break free from my cannulas and tubes so I could escape.

The seamless blurring of the boundaries between reality, thoughts, hallucinations and dreams was established right from the start. No matter how weird and implausible it seems now with hindsight, I believed everything to be real at the time. My memories of these are indistinguishable from those of events that actually did happen. My subconscious invented back stories, events and people. I clearly heard conversations between family member and nurses, which never happened, as my mind seemed to attempt to bring it all together and try to make some sort of sense of it all.

With hindsight some events were more obviously hallucinations – like the time a doctor came to talk to me, I couldn't listen to anything he was saying as I couldn't get beyond the fact that the ancient smart phone game of "snakes" (a short line of black pixels moving forward and turning though 90 degrees left and right) was playing out all over his crisp white shirt in 3D, all around his body, sleeves, collar, everywhere. Eventually, I would decide that, as a general rule, if I couldn't make out people's faces, I had probably made them up and possibly whatever else was happening at the time. Conversations would be going on slightly out of my field of vision – behind me, behind curtains, walls and partitions. Some hallucinations were very subtle, the room would be slightly different, in some the room was fine but I'd still make up clear conversations, some were bizarre beyond belief. I accepted everything without question, regardless.

Some of the encounters I'll never know if they actually happened. On one of these occasions, on my passage from ICU to HDU the general ward and returning back to ICU again, I arrived in a general ward which looked normal and as you would expect. I had a long conversation with a nurse who was about to end her shift. She came to sit with me and explained that she had had meningitis when she was around 18 months old. She obviously had no memories of her illness now, but was still living with the consequences and had some residual issues with anxiety and maintaining her concentration. Now a young mum herself with two children, she spoke of her own and her mother's worries during her pregnancies and while her children were young. I told her that I'd heard other nurses talking about me, my reputation had proceeded me, with my previous unruly behaviour and resisting the medication. She told me not to worry, she was very comforting and said that she would be back on duty in a couple of days and would look out for me. I was transferred again that day, so who knows?

That seemed to a bit of a theme, constantly moving between wards. I would always make a point of saying to the nurses, "Please ring my wife so she'll know which ward to visit". I made sure I'd slept before every visiting time, so I could recharge as fully as possible when she and other family members came to visit. I got to recognise her footsteps, I was always facing the door as she walk into the ward, it was the only guaranteed good part of every day, that all-so-easily-taken-for-granted pleasure of seeing a familiar face, when you only need just that. I know this seemed to contradict the subterfuge and the feeling of incarceration I had on other occasions, I somehow had at least two realities running simultaneously and I'd flip from one to the other.

Mostly the wards seemed to be laid out in a generally similar way, a series of six-bed open bays, three beds down each side along one side of a long corridor with the nurse's station, subsidiary rooms, cupboards and WCs along the other side. To me the first ward I was in, that I seemed to keep returning to, looked more like a

London Underground tube-station platform, the walls and vaulted roof covered in shiny white enamel brick-sized tiles. The beds were lined up along where the rails would have been and the corridor was along the platform. The beds were separated with pleated blue curtains between them, which also separated me from a treatment area behind me. The corridor area was always busy, noisy with people walking past. I did notice after a day or so that the same people seemed to walk past on several occasions and similar conversations were happening around me, which further confirmed my feeling of a deception going on all around me. Although the background, so to speak, seemed to be constant I do remember individual visits from doctors, nurses and family. The "actors" did on a few occasions, accidentally fall out of character and let things slip.

After I'd been discharged, I really struggled to make sense of the detail of what had actually happened, the chronological order of memories, events, and what was actually real. A day to day critical care diary referencing my medical notes was prepared for me by the wonderful ICU follow-up nurse Emma Madden as part of my aftercare.

On reflection, only in writing this, it's now becoming apparent that my mind seemed to have been compelling me to record what was happening, even while I was in hospital. When you'd think that would be the very last thing I should have been considering. It wasn't something I thought about, I just did it, almost in anticipation that at some point in the future I would need to put it all together to work out what had happened. Within the first day of being transferred from ICU to HDU, my first fully conscious day, I attempted to write about what I was thinking. Early on in the general ward stay I wrote notes on a leaflet to one of the disposable nebulisers I'd used, just recording events and dates. I heavy lined on it, in upper case "DO NOT THROW AWAY". Within the first week or two of being at home I wrote 11 pages of notes in an A5 notebook, while the memories were fresh in my mind. After my two months post discharge follow-up meeting I was fascinated by the critical care diary that was prepared, covering the period I was effectively unconscious. I also wanted to know from Trish, my wife, what had happened leading up to admission to hospital and the first weekend.

Initially I thought that my intention was to just put all this together and make sense of what happened to me while I was in hospital, but that has evolved into this.

What is to follow is based on all the information I have collated. This includes two WhatsApp threads my son and daughter used to disseminate news to the wider family and a group of friends, as well as subsequent conversations with my wife, children and friends. Also, how I saw and experienced events at the time.

Chapter Two

Early confusion, destination ICU

13 February 2016 (Saturday)

You came into the hospital with headache and confusion following a two-week history of a cough and sore throat.

While you were in A&E you had a CT scan, (computerised tomography scan using X-rays) of your head to find the cause of the headache and confusion. There was nothing abnormal detected on the scan.

You were admitted to Benham Ward where you had a lumbar puncture. A lumbar puncture is a medical procedure where a needle is inserted into the lower part of the spine to test for conditions affecting the brain, spinal cord or other parts of the nervous system.

The result of this came back as being bacterial meningitis. Meningitis is an infection of the protective membranes that surround the brain and spinal cord (meninges). You needed to be transferred to a side room to prevent cross infection with other patients, this was on Creaton Ward.

Truth is I'd had a chest infection for weeks before, I was okay-ish during the day but I was having difficulties breathing at night, so I took off-the-shelf medication which seemed to do the trick. I chose not to bother my GP with this, whether this somehow made me vulnerable for what was to follow, well who knows – probably not.

My last memories of Friday 12 February 2016 were of being in bed trying to get warm. I have no memories of events later that night, but seemed to have subsequently acquired a couple of vague isolated images of being in hospital, before I finally woke up in ICU around a week later.

By the time Trish came to bed I was apparently in some discomfort with a bad headache, she got me to take some paracetamol although this didn't seem to have any effect. She asked me if my headache was any better to which I responded, "No," but in a way she described as very unlike me, staring into space vague and emotionless.

She initially thought she would wait until the morning to see if I was any better, but my reaction to her played on her mind so much that she felt sure that there was something wrong. She became more concerned and asked if it was unlike any headache I'd had before, I said yes, but I stared right through her face blankly into the room beyond and then wouldn't speak at all. She became more worried and decided it couldn't wait and she rang 111. She was told by the operator to hold the phone to my ear so they could talk to me directly and they tried to get me to raise my arm and perform other tasks, I just didn't do anything and the operator said something like, "Mr Smith you must try to cooperate…"

Trish took the phone back saying, "There is something terribly wrong he's nonresponsive, you must send someone now." It was now in the early hours of Saturday and Trish was told to turn all the lights on in the house and look out for the ambulance which took about three hours to arrive. She spent this time alternating between pacing up and down the street outside the house and checking on me, particularly as I had vomited by this time. When the paramedics arrived and checked me out, they initially thought I may have had a stroke, but I became combative and apparently wasn't prepared to be taken willingly from my home and vigorously resisted. The landing and stairs were cleared of clutter and they strapped my arms and ankles to one of their chairs and carried me out struggling and holding on to the stair handrail whenever I could.

On arrival at hospital I was placed in A&E resuscitation, where I continued to appear vacant and wouldn't speak at all, only to curse now and again and generally show my reluctance to cooperate as I was being assessed by the doctors.

By now Trish had been joined by Gerri and Ken, her sister and brother-in-law. Trish had frantically been trying to contact our son and daughter but as it was Friday night into Saturday morning, neither of them responded to messages as they were recovering from their evenings out – as were other family members. My middle brother David, was woken early in the morning by my elder brother Paul, in South Africa on WhatsApp asking, "What on earth as happened to Pete?" Eventually they all made contact. David, and his partner Hazel, came to the hospital, along with our daughter Kate. And our son, George, came from Liverpool as soon as he could, later that weekend – what a star he'd matured into, he really stepped up to take control and support the family. He became the main contact for the hospital to take some pressure away from Trish and he kept the wider family informed, while Kate did the same fantastic job for a group of good friends in the village.

After being transferred to Benham Ward, to Trisha's shock and horror, I began to act like some drunk or a drug addict, which you might see on a medical documentary on the TV – cursing, behaving erratically. The doctor decided to do the lumber puncture but was convinced that I did not have mental capacity to consent to the procedure, to treatment or to understand what was going on. He immediately raised the necessary paperwork to withdraw the requirement to have my consent or Trisha's consent for what he felt was required.

Having a lumber puncture is apparently an uncomfortable procedure where you lie still on your side curled up to open the vertebrae of your back. The syringe needle can then more easily pass between the vertebrae so a sample of spinal fluid can be taken for analysis. After a rather hesitant nervous attempt by a young doctor, it was George that acted on what everyone else was thinking and got someone else to do it, the next guy did it like shelling peas, all over in a flash.

I was apparently restless during the procedure and occasional cursed at, well everyone in general. David and George helped to hold me down to the bed.

The possibility of meningitis was mentioned, and while the result was eagerly awaited a lot of googling went on, and then thoughts of, if it is that, then please let it be viral. The result promptly returned as meningococcal strain of bacterial meningitis. Trish watched one the doctors as he took the call at the nurses' station from the pathology lab, his face had a look of dismay. It was George who stood toe to toe, with me at one point, "Dad this has got serious now you've got to behave, get back in bed."

Which apparently, I duly did. I can't quite imagine what seeing someone you know so well acting so far out of character must have been like for everyone.

During the first weekend I was placed in the isolation room on a general ward as it was thought I might be contagious. Anyone with me was required to wear a surgical face mask, as I was still being assessed. I don't know the logistics of how it worked, but while still in hospital Trish receive a call on her cell phone from Public Health England, requesting details of anyone she'd had contact with during the previous 24 hours and were told that Kate and herself should collect a prescription for antibiotics, fetch them from the onsite pharmacy and take them straight away.

14 February 2016 (Sunday)

You had been started on antibiotics yesterday to treat the infection, but you still remain very confused and agitated.

Valentine's Day, around two months after I'd been discharged I suddenly remembered the card I'd written and put in a drawer in my desk ready to leave out for Trish, bit late that year.

15 February (Monday)

You were more settled in relation to your confusion today, but you could not remember the doctor who spoke to you in the morning. You were also unable to recall events that had happened since coming into hospital.

You developed a new left-sided facial droop and a left-eye squint with blurred vision. The doctor ordered another CT scan of your head as they were concerned about this.

You started to cough when you ate and the doctors were concerned about your swallow reflex. Your voice had become hoarse. A chest X-ray was performed to check if you had inhaled some food or drink. From now on, you were not allowed anything to eat or drink, you were Nil by Mouth (NBM).

The physio came to see you to help with some exercises to clear your chest.

In the evening you became very unwell. You developed a headache again, became very agitated and were short of breath. You had a blood test which showed your oxygen levels had dropped very low.

You were transferred to ICU.

As your oxygen levels were very low, the doctors put you to sleep (sedation) and put a breathing tube into your windpipe. We could then put you on a breathing machine (ventilator) so we could support your breathing and improve your oxygen levels. You had a feeding tube put into your nose that goes down to your stomach so we would be able to feed you while you are sedated.

You have a chest X-ray to confirm the tubes are in the right position. A drip is put into your arm that allows us to take blood regularly, and a large drip is put into your neck for us to give strong antibiotics through.

You are kept sedated.

The ICU/HDU period, approximately the first two weeks was uncompromisingly brutal, aggressive and left me utterly hollowed out. I was around two and a half stones lighter, almost 16kg. I had a left-side facial palsy, double vision, was incapable of shutting my left eye or of swallowing. I was also restricted in how wide I could open my jaw. The whole right-hand side of my body was numb from the top of my head to my toes. I was humbled and forced into to accepting, for the first time in my life, that I was incapable of anything physically or mentally. I became resigned to acquiesce completely and be totally reliant on those around me.

Fortunately, my brain switched off all cognitive functions for the first week when I wasn't sedated. So at the time I didn't remember removing the monitoring electrode contacts that were stuck to my chest, examining them and discarding them by apparently tossing them behind me over my shoulder, or pulling out the cannulas (needle and tube inserted into a vein or artery) from my wrists. They were "hidden" – wrapped in bandages in my ankles, I rubbed them so vigorously with my other foot the needle came out of the vein, but not my skin, this was discovered when someone looked under the sheet to find my foot had ballooned up tight as a drum. I had a large cannula stitched into my neck, I pulled it out and bloodied myself by scratching out every bit of the stitches. I seem to have acquired some very vague isolated images of doing this since.

I'd get up from bed and tangle the lines up. I resisted the administration of the powerful medication that was saving my life so forcefully, the hospital's security personnel were called in to hold me down. Trish said my arms and legs were black and blue with bruises and she was asked to leave the room while this was done. Very upsetting for my family, although my brother was told by a nurse it was actually an encouraging sign, she'd seen this a number of times during her career and those that fought strongly generally had a better chance of surviving and that I was very strong.

Not that I was consciously doing anything, but total war was being waged throughout my body between the overwhelming bacterial infection and the medication, with the medical team actively firefighting issues as they arose. The first was respiratory failure.

Trish, George, Kate, David and Hazel were visiting, and a nurse was with me. The oxygen level in my blood plummeted. Normally it should be between 94 per cent and 100 per cent, under 90 per cent is too low, under around 80 per cent for any length of time and all organs are being starved of oxygen and there is potential for permanent damage to them. Kate had been watching the monitor and said it dropped to 72 per cent. The red button was pushed and the nurse asked everyone to leave and wait outside the room. They were met by a rushing resuscitation team with trollies of equipment. They were all taken to the seminar room, where the staff made them a cup of tea as they were all in a state of shock. They were then taken the family room outside the ICU. After a couple of hours a doctor came into the room to tell them that I had been placed in an induced coma and put on a ventilator, she could not give them any further information but did advise that there was a possibility of brain or kidney damage as these organs are major oxygen consumers. They were allowed to visit me in ICU two at a time for a few minutes before they all left to go home. After two days Trish came in to sit with me as before and was told that at last my oxygen level had improved sufficiently to stop my sedation and I'd be allowed to wake up naturally. At this point they would be able to assess what "she'd been left with". Unfortunately, after several months, she concluded it was the same grumpy 50-something-year-old she'd become accustom to.

16 February (Tuesday)

You remain sedated today to allow the breathing machine to work at improving your oxygen levels

The microbiologist reviews the various blood and lumbar puncture results and starts you on some new antibiotics (you had been given some broad-spectrum antibiotics in A&E).

The dietician reviews you and prescribes a liquid feed we can give you through your feeding tube.

Medical note indicated: Sepsis develops

Discharge summary indicated: intubated in ICU and perri-arrest

The peri-arrest period is the recognised stage, either just before or just after a full cardiac arrest, when the patient's condition is very unstable and care must be taken to prevent progression or regression into a full cardiac arrest. Fortunately, sufficient intervention successfully prevented full cardiac arrest from developing.

---

17 February (Wednesday)

The neurologist team reviewed your results: they have nothing new to add to your current treatment.

Your sedation was stopped and you wake up enough for your breathing tube to come out at night. Your breathing is more settled and your oxygen levels have improved.

Being woken from sedation, for me, didn't involve the gradual, gentle way that happens when you wake from a normal sleep in somewhere you know with a stretch and yawn. You're not actually asleep and don't achieve the regenerative sleep that is needed. It's like flicking a switch on and off, blinking, the eyes open and you're there, somewhere unrecognisable for however long it takes to complete whatever task or procedure is needed. You're not aware of being put back to sleep, only the same waking process where your eyes open again and you're maybe in a different room with different people. There may have been minutes, hours or days between but, with the blink of the eye, the whole scene and everyone in it changes. And I'd no idea why any of it was happening at all.

18 February (Thursday)

You are seen by the Speech and Language Team (SALT). They are unhappy with your swallow reflex, and say you are unable to eat or drink. You continue to have the liquid diet through your feeding tube.

19 February (Friday)

You have a neurological examination, which shows you have left-sided facial nerve palsy. Bell's palsy is a weakness that affects the muscles of the face. It develops suddenly, usually on one side of the face. The cause is not clear but most cases are probably due to a viral infection. Most people make a full recovery within two to three months.

I am still waiting for the two to three months to start.

It was Kate, who noticed my facial palsy first. Which, it transpires, is a result of damage to my seventh cranial nerve, which should control some muscles for facial expression and taste sensations to a fairly large portion of my tongue.

20 February (Saturday)

You are more stable, and do not require the support of the intensive doctors now, so you are transferred to Benham Ward

21 February (Sunday)

A member of the Critical Care Outreach team visits you on the ward to review your observations and blood results. You have a swollen abdomen and had not had your bowels open for more than seven days. You have an ultrasound of your abdomen and are started on some laxatives and enemas to resolve this.

The less said about that the better.

22 February (Monday)

You are given a patch to wear over your eye, and some drops to put in it, as due to the muscle weakness in your face, the eye can become very dry. SALT gives you some jaw exercises to do. You have been transferred to Becket Ward.

I couldn't blink or shut my left eye so it became very dry and ointment was applied regularly to help with this. Also, for some reason I had developed double vision. The patch over one eye blocked one image so what I was seeing looked a bit more normal. I'd swap the patch over eye to eye now and again. Without it I saw a perfect double image side by side. Faces were almost twice the width with four perfect eyes in a line and two noses side by side in the most convincing Photoshop I'd seen. This lasted for 10 days. I had noted on the leaflet that on 3 March I woke up and looked at the clock on the wall opposite, it was round again instead of the horizontal figure of eight I was becoming used to, I was also able to read much more easily.

23 February (Tuesday)

SALT review you again. They feel your swallow reflex is improving; however it is inconsistent and therefore you remain NBM.

You become very short of breath, and are unable to talk in full sentences, indicating you are finding your breathing very hard. Again, your oxygen levels are low, but this time you do not need the breathing tube to help improve them.

You have developed pneumonia. You are given some "high flow" oxygen which helps increase your levels.

You have blood cultures taken and are started on new anti-biotics as the doctors think you are suffering from sepsis. Sepsis, also referred to as blood poisoning or septicaemia, is a potentially life-threating condition, triggered by an infection or injury. In sepsis, the body's immune system goes into overdrive as it tries to fight an infection.

Sepsis can't be caught, it's not contagious and does not remain within you, although resulting issues may do. Normally our immune system fights infection – but sometimes, for reasons not yet fully understood, it attacks our body's own organs and tissues. If not treated immediately, sepsis can result in multiple organ failure and death.

Prompt diagnosis and treatment is crucial as the progression can be rapid, after diagnosis it thought that every hour delay in treatment can increases the chance of death by seven and a half percent. There are around 250,000 cases a year in the UK, approximately 55,000 are fatal, just over one in five. One in four of those that survive will have permanent life changing effects. Sepsis kills more people in the UK than lung cancer or bowel cancer, breast cancer and prostate cancer combined

---

This time, for approximately nine days, my oxygen was delivered via an oxygen nasal cannula, which is a tube hung around my ears and passing under my nose with a horn projecting up each nostril. This was attached to a steel oxygen canister which became my buddy as I was moved around the hospital in the bed to a different ward, or in the wheelchair to various departments.

I never seemed to get all the pipework on my nose comfortable and it needed constant adjustment. The oxygen tube rubbed the rim of my ears red and sore and the pointed horns would either rub the inside of my nose or flip out. The nasogastric (NG) feeding tube was held in place with a piece of sticky tape. I spent hours trying to invent, in my head, a simple comfortable alternative to do the job of attaching the oxygen tube and the NG feeding tube to my nose. Once I'd cracked this, I could imagine nurses everywhere at some point saying to each other, right patient X needs a "Smith", nip over and get one from supplies, how did we ever manage without one of these? Never a dull moment.

Chapter Three

24 to 25 February –
total train crash

24 February (Wednesday)

You are transferred back to ICU where you have a tight-fitting face mask to give you oxygen under pressure. Your heart goes into a very fast irregular rhythm. This may be due to the strain and overwhelming infection your body is suffering from.

Medical notes indicate: Type 1 Respiratory failure.

There are eight beds in HDU and eight beds in ICU, one of which is in a room on its own, this is where I am now. It's a typical hospital room, bare neutral painted walls, squared suspended tile ceiling, windowless and loads of equipment. There is one double door for access. This is where the above procedure is being done, having first been bought out of sedation. The mask is like a diving mask that fits over your eyes, nose and mouth, it has a hose connected at the bottom where warm moist air/steam is pumped in. At the time I was semi-conscious and hallucinating very badly, so my experience of the procedure and how it felt to me was rather different to the reality. I'd been carried on a stretcher down a spiral staircase that followed the long curve of the wall into this dimly lit circular dungeon and placed on my back on a central bed. I don't remember having anything explained to me about what was about to happen, but also knew I wouldn't have the strength to resist it either. I somehow knew it needed to be done, so deep breath, man up, and just take whatever is coming. It felt as though I was being held down to the bed while at least two other people were watching from the stairs. My head was shaken around as the mask was being fitted, much like a busy parent would do to put a nappy on a restless baby. One other person was sitting on my pelvis, astride me and was using their whole-body weight to force an air-tight fit of the mask to my face, pushing my head into the pillow. The hose channelled a pressured warm mist of moist oxygen into the mask which quickly filled, steamed up the glass and spilled into my eyes, nose and mouth, and mixed with that distinctive smell of warmed rubber and plastic. This made breathing naturally and smoothly impossible, it felt as though a constant "in" pressure was working against my laboured in out breathing, and that I was competing, and losing, against the machine to breath at all. I could only manage irregular snatched short sharp intakes of breath as I felt the corner of my eyes oozing with tears of discomfort. Like a mist rolling over a moorland landscape, I could feel the warmth roll through me all the way down to my lungs, it's a strange feeling being warmed from the inside. The mask was only briefly removed so I could cough up/vomit phlegm into a bowl, the process was then repeated until there was nothing left to cough up, don't know if this was the purpose of the procedure or an unfortunate consequence. This all took a lot of time and finished late into the night, too late to return to a ward.

When this procedure was completed, I was moved to another part of the hospital through a network of Victorian brick-walled and vaulted corridors beneath the hospital that are used to move patients around the building more efficiently. Sometimes the nurses pushed me around on a trolley (as happened this time). On other occasions I was strapped in a strait jacket to a trolley that ran on small gauge rails, this was automated so you could be sent around the building as required. A bit like a larger version of the Victorian shop/ department store tube system for moving cash and receipts around from the shop floor to a backroom office. I watched the lengths of ceiling strip lights slowly pass by if I was being pushed along or flash by, strobe-like and faster if I was on the rails.

Anyway, that night I was transferred to an overnight holding area with several others, we were all supposed to be sedated. I was still semi-conscious and could clearly hear the conversation of the nurses chatting as they transferred me through the tunnel system. To save space (I know its madness) we were all secured in sleeping bag type cocoons and with a system of pulleys raised up and hung on a tall wall like bats in a cave. In case we woke up, to give the illusion that we were lying down, there was a table and chairs and a clock fixed on the wall opposite me, they were rotated through 90 degrees if you were standing on the floor upright, but looked the right way viewed from where we were hanging. I was so disorientated and dizzy that it took me a while and some concentration to work out which way up I was and I still got it wrong. Periodically a nurse would check on us to make sure we were okay. I was still wearing the mask from the procedure, which was still full of the warm steamy air. Having broken the seal to check on me the rapid change in temperature and air pressure was enough to wake me from the semi-sedation and I coughed. I remember the conversation I had with the nurse, they still couldn't move me to the ward and I was comfortable at the time, so I was left to rest or sleep there. After such an eventful evening, finally being left alone was a very welcomed break, even though I was still restrained in a strait jacket, such a relaxed deep sense of calm washed over me. There was a window close by to my left side through which I could see the nightscape of the town. I was high up and had an elevated view down on to the streets. They were empty, quiet, peaceful, dark and wet – it had been raining. I could see the pools of light in puddles reflected from an array of amber streetlights and traffic lights slowly changing. I saw buildings I recognised, the lower parts of the general hospital sprawled out in the foreground, the Carlsberg brewery and the rest of the town beyond with a partially cloud filled blue dark night sky. As day broke the nurse came back to check on me again. She told me that she had reported what had happen, it was apparently very rare to make such a rapid recovery form the procedure and I was expected do a live television interview on Spanish breakfast TV. I do remember thinking even in my delusion, this was grossly unfair, why was I required to do this although I couldn't see all my family. After careful consideration and a few attempts at persuasion from the NGH management, I declined and I assume the waiting presenter and film crew where sent back to Spain.

I didn't know how long after the procedure it was, but remember being awake, on planet Earth, in a normal room and feeling quite good, feeling this was the low point that had passed. I asked the nurse if I could have the mask as a souvenir, I was told these were single use and would usually be destroyed, but why not? They must have thought this was a bit bizarre. I still have it in a bag at home. Trish hates it, so it has to stay hidden away.

I was terribly wrong; my decline would continue for a while longer.

On 19 May 2017, I met one of my ICU nurses for the first time, Nurse A, who remembered that she was with me during the mask procedure. This was at an event celebrating 50 years of critical care at NGH, that I was invited to attend. It was particularly rewarding for me as I was able to talk to her and thank her. It was an afternoon tea for previous patients, their family and staff – the staff celebrated a little more vigorously in the evening. It was very well attended, a lovely afternoon. ICU is a particularly unique and challenging nursing position. Constant one-to-one nursing and they don't normally get to see their patients walk out of the Unit better, only moved on as they are stepped down to a general ward. As patients are generally sedated while in their care the nurse and patient don't get to know each other and of course the Unit's mortality rate, by its very nature, must be relatively high. So the nurses are constantly seeing very worried, upset or bereaved family members. We sat and had a cup of tea together and chatted almost like old friends. The bond you feel on such occasions really is like nothing else, I've experienced this now a few times. I was talking with her for the first time, but knowing she had spent 12-hour shifts one-to-one monitoring and caring for me when I was at my most vulnerable. It truly is a debt you can never adequately repay. I decided to explain what the procedure felt like for me, absolutely horrified just about sums up how she felt. But I forgave her and we hugged and made up.

25 February (Thursday)

Your heart is still in the very fast and irregular rhythm. The doctor's give you a controlled electric shock to bring it back to a normal speed and rhythm.

I didn't know these two procedures were so close together until I'd read my medical notes sometime after.

I had already suffered type 1 respiratory failure and had a peri cardiac arrest. I now still had meningococcal bacterial meningitis, sepsis, pneumonia, and my heart rate had been averaging 170 beats per minute since sometime the previous day.

I'm woken from my sedation. I'm still in the room with one bed and inexplicitly, more conscious and aware right now than I've been since arriving in hospital. Although I have this strange feeling of almost detachment from the scene as though I'm viewing myself in a virtual reality. I can't remember at any point actually being told "Mr Smith you are ill" so this can't actually be happening. Initially it felt as if I was being emotionally drawn into a very realistic, compelling video game in which, if it went badly wrong, a restart button could be pressed. The room has a number of people in it who all seem to be standing over me, I don't recognise any of them so overwhelmingly the feeling I have is of vulnerability and being alone. I can do nothing to influence whatever is going to be done to me, I don't know why it's needed or what has happened.

I'm on a bed with the head end slightly raised to enable the feeding tube to work by gravity. I am now feeling very weak. It's not just the speed my heart is beating, around three times a second, it's the strength of the pounding, I feel my whole torso moving in sync with it. I can see the display of the monitor that I'm connected to, it appears to be randomly generating numbers between just under 160 and the mid-180s. The main man is standing by my left knee and he's talking to a small group of people in white coats around my right foot. He is using words and phrases I just don't understand for the most part, but then something like "but this can be temporarily controlled by," and I see this hand move down to somewhere near the left side of my neck. I can't feel anything at all, but pretty much straight away I feel my heart slowing to a stop, and my eyelids are so heavy I can't keep them open.

He stopped whatever he was doing, and my eyes opened again. In no more than a handful seconds my heart rate went from around 180 beats per minute to zero and back to 180 again. I think he said something like, "That shouldn't be happening as quickly as that."

The atmosphere dramatically changed, darkened. I'm sure he'd assumed the waving gestures of his hand low down close to his thighs was out of my field of view as he spoke, again things I didn't understand. Instantly the people at my right foot were gone and a nurse appeared each side of me, I watched them as they got busy installing additional cannulas to those I already had in both wrists. While this was going on, I had eye contact with the main man, this was my first involvement in what was happening, so it now became alarming very real, an overused word, but I experienced my first genuine feelings of fear. He spoke directly to me. "Your heart rate is averaging 170 beats per minute, this is just not sustainable, at that rate its consuming muscle as an energy source. We must give you a controlled electric shock to bring it back under control. We'll do this while you are sedated. We'll sedate you, perform the procedure and then bring you around again. The whole process will take no more than around eight seconds. We're putting additional cannulas into your wrists, this is nothing for you to be concerned about, if any stage of this procedure does not go precisely as I've planned, I want all options open to me immediately. When you come around your chest may hurt, but again this would be completely normal and nothing for you to be concerned about."

I was sort of expecting a countdown but this didn't come, in fact I only just had time to roll my eyes up to the ceiling and think, *that will be the last thing I'll ever see.*

Incredibly, for me the eight seconds took less than one, it was almost like the continuation of the same sentence. "And you're back."

There was some activity around me but the atmosphere lightened quickly. I looked over to the monitor, the display was now reading between mid-90s and just over 100 and the room seemed to almost empty quickly. I was left with a nurse who was busying herself, getting rid of stuff and generally tiding up. There's a long awkward silence that I eventually chose to break, by saying the stupidest thing, "Pity that wasn't recorded I would have liked to see that."

Without looking up from what she was doing, the nurse said,

"No, you wouldn't, we have to for our training, it's horrible." I blinked (although I was sedated) I've no idea how long after the event this was and I think I was in the same room. The nurse was gone and the main man had reappeared to examine me and asked some questions, he seemed general happy with the result of his, and his team's work. As he flipped off his blue latex gloves, he finished by asking if I smoked, "No," I said.

"Probably just as well, had you been a smoker, overweight or just generally not as fit as you clearly were, that might well have turned out differently," with that I was knocked out again.

My heart rate at rest remained at between 100 and 105 beats per minute for around four months, then gradually over the next three months or so finally calmed down to a healthy 60 to 70, where it's been since. I've also learnt since (googled), that in the condition I was in, if the heart rate goes a bit wild, it can sometimes just as randomly sort itself out, and can be left as it is. It's a judgement call on the likelihood of that happening, against the relative strength of the patient at that time, and what that is likely to be if it is left any longer. I used to think I made big decisions once. Everything I saw that day was so impressive, like a Formula 1 racing team pit crew, everything being done to an accurate plan, professionally, very quickly, efficiently but without any sense of panic. I suppose it's all relative, but I just don't think the same way now.

It's pretty extraordinary what etches permanently into your brain with so little contact. These were the only moments I saw the main man at the time. Around eight months later, on 2 November 2016, as part of the NGH Sepsis Awareness Week, the in-house magazine ran an article about it and I was asked if I'd do a patient interview account/story, of course I was very happy to oblige. The main part of the article was by the appropriate consultant and included a photograph of him. When I saw it for the first time, I instantly recognised him. It was also the corroboration I needed. Now I have the mask and I have him, sorted.

It was these brief few moments that I thought of so often and so much about at the time, afterwards and occasionally ever since. Why was this brief period the one in which I was the most aware and lucid? And how, from being sitting at home apparently fit and healthy, twelve days later did I find myself here?

I was fortunate enough to meet the main man again almost three years later, on 6 February 2019, at a Sepsis Roadshow Awareness Day that I'd been invited to attend, a joint event between The Sepsis Trust, NGH and Northampton University. I was busy at the buffet table loading my plate with free sandwiches, I looked up and he was directly opposite me doing the same, I could see he actually recognised me. I took this opportunity to briefly talk to him, shake his hand and thank him. He told me that he had massaged a collection of nerve ending at the left side of my neck, this is known as a Carotid Massage. This procedure had unintentionally, unfortunately caused my heart to briefly stop. He also confirmed that the follow up, check-up consultation would have been the day after the procedure. Initially I was rather surprised that he recognised me, I thought it must be my resemblance to George Clooney or must have made an impression somehow, but discovered the sepsis article from the magazine was reproduced as a poster and was put up all round the hospital, it was still in the lift outside ICU, so he'd probably shared the lift with me most days.

At a tea break I also managed to have a conversation with a speaker at this event, the head of the Pathology department at NGH, after a while he asked how I'd acquired my sepsis.

"I had bacterial meningitis."

"Do you know what particular strain of the bacteria it was?" "Meningococcal."

"You had meningococcal septicaemia," he said, with an alarming look of surprise on his face. I was a bit confused as I hadn't heard what I had described in that way before "… err… yes."

He said he'd like to continue our chat and invited me to make an appointment and accompany him on a tour of the Pathology department. I initially thought of this in the same way you do when on holiday and you have a brilliant time with someone you haven't met before and say we must meet up when we get home, of course you never do. But he mentioned it again as the event was finishing, explaining that, normally he wouldn't see the results of this work or meet the patients and would like to talk further about my apparent good recovery from the infection. I couldn't refuse really, what an amazing opportunity.

The day came, 12 February 2019, and first we sat around the conference table in his office and chatted over a cup of tea. The lumber puncture procedure came up in the conversation and he said that he would show me where my sample would have been analysed. I was given a visitor's white lab coat and we commenced an amazing hour-long tour of the department – unbelievable.

I walked past a conveyer belt full of thousands of files of blood samples from the wards and elsewhere passing through automated machines, robot arms swinging around to select individual samples to test and recording each one. And apparently having the results on the system to be accessed anywhere within the hospital within 20 minutes of arriving. We moved from specialist room to specialist room, watching biopsies, cultures and sample slides being prepared for analysis. I had what was going on in there explained to me and being politely introduced each time we met someone as "Mr Smith who has survived meningococcal disease", then watching raised eyebrows of surprise appear around the room. Information overload set in, I kept my hands in my pockets and daren't breathe or cough for fear of contaminating something. Eventually we arrived at the room where the lumber puncture samples are tested and I was allowed to sit with the technician as she worked at the station with the equipment that would have been used to test my sample. She tried to explain what she was doing to me in a way that I might understand and did retrieve an image of the meningococcal bacteria for me to look at. I regrouped enough to think *I'll never be able to repeat this visit and can't leave without asking the big question.* "How many times would you expect to see this infection in… let's say a year?"

After a considered pause the answer came, "Three or four."

We completed the tour and arrived back at his office, with me in a slight state of shock, another cup of tea and a relaxed chat to regroup again and address the elephant in the room.

"If you were to see this infection three or four times in a year, how many of these people would you expect to survive?"

"If I saw it five times in a year… none… or maybe one. You need to understand the nature and progression of this infection. These bacteria can survive harmlessly on the surface of the skin for weeks, possibly up your nose just waiting for a way into your bloodstream, any tiny cut or graze. Once it's entered your bloodstream, if left untreated its almost always fatal, you have between two and four days left. It progresses to a stage…"

He gave that a name and acronym that I can't remember now. This is on day one or two of the infection, when it then begins to break down the bodies cell walls.

He continued, "Having reached this point, the situation is irretrievable and you have one or two days left. In fact, had you already progressed to this stage when you were admitted here, we would, of course, thrown everything we have at you, but there wouldn't have been a realistic prospect of you surviving. I've seen this when I've worked in poorer countries in Africa that simply don't have the resources we have here, infants typically may not survive the day. Survivors can quite commonly lose limbs or extremities, have epilepsy or any number of other life altering deficits. So, if I looked surprised when we met as you were standing in front of me apparently healthy, it's because I was. Your wife did exactly the right thing in getting you here promptly, you must get started on antibiotics as early as possible."

It's peculiar to think that having spoken to the lab technicians, before they met me, three or four times a year, when they see this infection they couldn't help but to think that if the person this sample came from isn't already dead, they probably will be in a couple of days' time. Now they may think that this person could survive.

A meningococcal infection doesn't always lead to sepsis or other complications, and if treated early enough, mortality rate can drop from around 90 to 95 per cent to around 15 per cent.

Chapter Four

Finally, on the way back

26 February (Friday)

You are more stable and are moved through to the HDU. You have a chest X-ray, which shows you still have pneumonia and a repeat abdominal ultrasound, this is normal.

From this day on, although still a bit bonkers for a while, finally every new day, was actually an improvement on the previous one, although it didn't necessarily feel like it to me at the time. It's a curious thing being critically ill through an infection and the complications that ensue, rather than some sort of physical injury. Although every part of my body and mind was mercilessly under attack, I felt very little pain. Whether I was awake, dreaming or hallucinating the only difference was in what I was experiencing, so there was nothing to anchor a perception of which particular state I was in. Had I been in pain, might that be changed or removed when I was dreaming or hallucinating, who knows?

Improving was only the case in the real world, when I flipped to an alternative reality I'd only progressed from not being ill at all and needing to escape, to accepting that everyone genuinely thought I was ill and having to convince them I was improving by acting out a recovery, so someday I could bluff my way out of there. Or being terminally ill and being transferred to a hospice that was attached to the hospital. It was very confusing, experiencing and believing all that at various stages and then clearly overhearing conversations between hospital staff or staff and family members corroborating it.

This second period, the third week, was frightening. Although up to that point I was either sedated or my brain was protecting me from experiencing some of what I was happening. I didn't know this was a temporary holding exercise and it'd all come out, and have to be dealt with, starting at around three months after I was discharged, after the "holiday period". However, from now, I was aware of everything that was happening but wasn't aware I was also hallucinating, and/or having very vivid dreams and seemed to be incapable of differentiating between these states.

Having been transferred to HDU, I wasn't sedated again. This started the precarious transition between times of being aware, lucid and periods of constant insanity and slipping back into my bad behaviour. Sometimes when I felt more aware, I knew that I'd only need the wrong dream/experience and I'd revert back into the weird world.

At least being awake a lot of the time I was able to chat more with the nurses, I remember after Trish, George and Kate left at the end of the afternoon visiting time in HDU my nurse made a point of saying to me, "That must be your son, what an impressive young man, the way he behaves here and looks after and comforts his mum, absolutely wonderful to see, you should be so proud of him."

I think it was around this time, in a parallel universe, I was transferred to a larger ward which had more beds in and seemed to be like something from the 1950s, with high ceilings. The nurse's uniforms were more old fashioned, blue with white aprons, pristine starched white folded headwear. There was a distinct philosophical difference between, two very different groups of nurses here, the usual NHS nurses and a group I can only describe as like the Christian Brethren or Amish people of North America. This ward seemed to be a sort of halfway house between the "normal" hospital and the hospice where I was destined to end up. Also, the place in which members, including the elders of the group would be cared for away from the general public taking account of their particular religious believes and customs, instead of being in the normal hospital wards. There was another "non-believer" like me on the opposite side a little further down the ward from me. I eavesdropped as he was sitting on his bed with his back to me, on his mobile phone trying to explain what this environment was like to someone, he ending up saying that is was "kind of nice, comforting really".

To comfort, console and reaffirm the beliefs of this group, their nurses would spend time talking with them. Their nurse would occasionally lie on top of the bed with those that were terminally ill to spiritually comfort them or if they were struggling emotionally with their illness or recovery. They would read from, debate and discuss their particular scriptures.

In preparation for each evening there was almost a sort role reversal between the higher ranking elder and the nurses. The nurses took more of a dominant controlling, supporting role to ensure they did as they were required, ensuring their recovery was kept on track. For those that were more mobile, they'd take part in some sort of team game in the room next door to this ward. I clearly heard an ice hockey puck like object sliding across a hard floor and hitting into a steel frame which I took to being a goal. When I finally began to walk, I actually made a point of looking behind the wall to check how the room was laid out, it surprisingly turned out to be just another ward bay of six beds.

After a while I was transferred to what I'd assumed was the hospice, this was staffed completely with the "Brethern" nurses. I was taken into a room with one bed, it was quite attractive with sunlight streaming through an open French door with thin net curtains waving in a breeze. Rather spookily the bed was made up with a stiff starched sheet folded and formed origami style in a recognisable shape of one of the nurses with bonnet type headwear. I took this to mean as a non-believer I didn't warrant an actual person and it was genuinely meant as some sort of comfort for my last days. I got rid of that off the bed pretty damn quick. As I settled into my bed, I could hear a group of people laughing and chatting, listening and relaxing to a music concert in the garden area outside, singing along to songs I didn't recognise. This was out of my field of vision through the window, and I definitely got the impression this was for others to appreciate, I wasn't to be included.

I didn't like this place, it had the atmosphere – the smell of a place that you never walked out of. I remember ringing Trish imploring her to get me transferred out of there.

Trish and Kate did visit me there on one occasion, I could hear them behind the wall as though they were in a corridor area, but they seemed to pass by on a number of occasions as though their route was for some reason artificially extended. This must have slightly frustrated them as I heard them express a little displeasure regarding this. I then heard them being chastised about this and they had to then to wait and reflect on things before they were allowed to come through to see me. I questioned Trish about this when the eventually arrived at my bedside, she was rather confused.

27 and 28 February

You are less confused and your condition is more stable.

During this transition period, alternating between bad behaviour/good patient, with not much else to do or think about, I became very preoccupied and obsessive about the NG tube and my feeding. Such a simple thing, the tube was either, unnecessarily fixing me to the bed and had to be removed, so I would pull it out to enable me to escape, or it was a major anxiety when it wasn't there because I would starve. When I was more rational and got a little more mobile, for instance when I began to stand up to wash in the morning, it would slip out. Not much consistent logical thought going on at the time and just one of the many contradictions I struggled with. I had many weird, what turned out to be, surreal dreams about this.

Replacing the NG tube was really uncomfortable. The procedure is to measure with the tube, from the tip of the nose along the cheek to the neck then down the neck to just below your chest to approximately where the stomach is, (62cm for me). Then feed it though the nostril, until the end reached the muscly flappy bit that hinges to either cover the opening to your lungs or stomach, depending on if you're breathing or swallowing. Then a pause, and a synchronised swallow and a push on the tube to take it down in to the stomach, fine, unless the flappy bit doesn't work, then all the nurse can do is poke and jab until it forces its way through. If this didn't work a stiffer tube was used which had a wire through it that could be withdrawn when it was in place. To check it was in the stomach rather than the lungs some icky fluid is drawn up and acid/alkaline tested and compared against a colour chart. If this was inconclusive a chest X-ray had to be done to verify it's in the correct position and a piece of tape was used to attach it to the end of my nose. This happen almost every day that I was conscious, (either self-inflected or accidentally) sometimes two or three times a day.

During this period, I did have significant anxieties about what the night might bring. As the lights dimmed for bedtime, I'd raise my head and allow it drop to the pillow, repeating the mantra in my head, *I am in the right place, I am ill, no one is here to harm me, stop fucking about.* Hoping it would just lodge somewhere and I'd behave all night. It didn't work all the time and as I drifted off to sleep sometimes a handful of images played through my mind and drew me into the weird world. I had this recurring dream. The scene didn't develop fully but kept replaying over and over again. These images were initially pretty innocuous in themselves and looked sort of familiar. Eventually I convinced myself they were based on photos on my previous phone which was unused in a drawer at home, as long as they existed this simply would not stop. Those photos had to be deleted. I somehow managed to persuade Trish to take a break and get a cup of tea so that I could get some time alone with my daughter Kate during the afternoon visit. I told her it was important and I made her promise that when she got home to find the phone, charge it up and delete every photo on it. That night the same scenes replayed again, but then it got weirder. It was like I was inside the phone's memory lying down on my back on a platform that moved very fast, stopping and starting instantly and in all directions in a vast dimly lit enclosed space, briefly pausing by a lightened panel that then went out, before racing off to find another, so fast and real I started to feel nauseous as this played out for ages. I didn't get that dream again afterwards. Nothing to do with the photos of course but says a lot about the faith I had in my 20-year-old daughter doing what I'd asked her to, yes that how deluded I was.

I only had one recurring upsetting nightmare which thankfully eventually stopped as the medication finally began to be reduced.

There was one evening in particular when I must have been in HDU that stands out from all the others during the whole time I was in hospital. For no reason that was obvious to me, I felt very powerfully that I simply would not wake up the next morning. It wasn't a case of thinking I wouldn't, I absolutely knew this was beyond any doubt. At the end of the evening visiting time, Trish was in the process of tidying things and making sure I had everything I needed close by before she left. As she was doing this, I had two very clear voices in my head, *"You need to say goodbye,"* then, *"Too dramatic you drama queen,"* then, *"Well if you don't do it now, things will never get said, you won't get another opportunity."*

So, I did, we spoke, kissed and she left. With hindsight, on top of everything else Trish had to cope with this can't have helped, particularly as on two occasions it had been suggested to her that it might be a good idea if she prepared herself for whatever the outcome might be. I can't remember what was going through my mind as I lay there deep into that night, but a ward full of people can be a very lonely place. As I got more tired, when I felt my eyes closing and could feel myself falling asleep, I'd rock my head from side to side or lift it up a little and let it drop to the pillow, consciously breathe erratically, quickly force my eyes wide open, anything I could think of to stop the sleep. I don't know how long I managed this but inevitably I got to the point where sleeping was unstoppable. I'd just run out of strength. With a real sense of, I have nothing left and resignation, I spoke to myself, *"Stopping the sleep isn't going to change anything, it isn't going to make me well, what will happen, will happen… "* so I had to let go and let it happen. Knowing that when my eyes shut my life was over.

One little known fact about the HDU bay I was in, was that it periodical detached from the building slid down a ramp and "Thunderbirds-style" attached to an articulated lorry and, along with several others, toured the county in some sort of help, outreach programme, visiting schools and drop-in medical centres. I was demoted to skivvy because of my unruly behaviour. This also meant my incarceration was prolonged; I had to fully serve my time. On one of these trips, at lunchtime I had a long in-depth conversation with a total stranger about the injustice being done to me, my conniving family and what I should do about it. After years in a marriage with a controlling husband she'd final got divorced and never felt happier. She was very sympathetic and completely agreed with me, so I must be right.

I napped frequently during the day, but one particular evening and long into the night, I remember seeing a guy just sitting in a chair, a little away from me outside the open cubical I was in, just sitting there doing nothing. I fell asleep and woke up a little later he was still there, fell asleep, woke up, still there on and on all night. I only remembered this months later at home and at one of my many deep low points in recovery joking moaned, NHS wastage blah blah. Trish told me, that night the one nurse to two patients in HDU wasn't enough, there was such concern for my wellbeing and an agency nurse was brought in just to keep an eye on me.

As part of the dealing with this whole experience much later, I only had one, what I'd call a flashback and that only happened the once. I didn't work at all for around two months after I was discharged. I was then able to gradually build-up and do short sessions and then rest. With hindsight I did too much too soon and things quickly built and I put myself under a bit of pressure. I did what I'd been used to doing for years, if things got a little out of control. Give up on the digital to-do list and hand write a list in pencil of the most urgent items, most pressing at the top, allocate a sensible time frame, then ring the various clients first before they rang to chase me, and give them the revised good/bad news. I've always been of the opinion that the best form of defence is attack. Then do the tasks in order and rub them out one at a time. I choose to get out of the house and get some space to do this. I took a pad and pencil and drove into the countryside, parked up in field gateway the middle of nowhere, it happened as soon as my pencil touched the paper, bang. I had escaped from my hospital bed but was wrestling resisting, struggling with some people but quickly tired and was put on a trolley. The room looked like a foyer type area with almost a reception type desk possibly a ward nurses' station as there were two nurses sitting behind it. Some of the walls were exposed facing brickwork. I tried to get back up again but only managed to get on to my hands and knees on the trolley which then felt precarious. I was so very weak and thought if I fell from here I wouldn't have the strength to get back up again, my head dropped and I looked down between my supporting arms, all the cannulas were gone from my wrists and my forearms were covered in blood. I managed to turn around and lie back down. As I lay there exhausted, I started remembering previous events which all seem disconnected and didn't make sense. I asked the nurses for some paper and a pen, which they fetched and pushed the tray table over me. I starting writing bullet points down, things that I felt were significant, to try and put some order to it and to see if things did connect in some way. My hand moved slowly and awkwardly. I could barely read the couple of lines I managed. I let the paper fall to the floor and started again concentrating on trying to write legibly. It ended there, I don't know what happened after that, but it just stopped. I didn't know if it was because I'd fell asleep or because I'd woken up.

I sorted myself out, started the car and drove home. Couldn't wait to get inside the house, Trish was sat on the sofa watching the TV. I told her all about it, this messed up weird flashback/dream or whatever I'd had. First thing she said was "I have the piece of paper."

Trish had come in to see me as usual one day, and was shocked at the state of me, I looked unwashed, dirty, dishevelled, black fingernails, a right mess. She spoke to the nurse, who said they'd done their best to clean me up but I'd been a total nightmare that night, uncontrollable, the black under my nails was dry blood. Trish saw a piece of paper on the cupboard at the side of my bed, recognised the writing as mine but could only make out the odd word and couldn't understand any of it. She folded it up and put in in her bag. When she got home, she put it in the draw in our bedside cabinet. There it was some five months later. I couldn't bring myself to try and read it, I wasn't ready then, so there it stopped untouched for another six months until January 2017. I remembered it and reading it felt right.

Typical engineer I'd dated the paper, it was 27 February 2016, I had just been moved from ICU to HDU and relinquished the one-to-one nursing of ICU and had to share my nurse with one other patient.

27/FEB 16.

duty is Triste ~~& my~~ ^(ME with) relationship is ~~The~~
there our ~~too~~ under arrest. do the

Why do we ~~sleep~~ in a ~~define~~ t
this, where do we ~~both~~ ~~lye~~ live, wh
ONLY SEEM NOT ~~KNOW~~ KNOW. ~~WHY~~ v
~~about~~ WE MOVE BE TROGETER or
MY SA STORY ~~&~~ VISION OF OUR

WHY SCOULDN'T WE DEVORCE.
~~I~~ ROTORED IT, WHY DONT I KNOW
HOW LON
WHAT HAVE I DO NEXT,
~~regi~~ getting ~~fumalyle~~ Fies to too b
Dove & Hazol?
Pout.   why didnt

HAVE I ~~HEEPED~~ over-protection isse
~~Ball~~ ~~some~~ of my ~~conflict~~ allegations
clearing colour
what is not

50

IT SEEMS
IS,.. HAVE I done anything illegal are
know... why do not relate at all!
know long a miss beeth
why have sthethings been developed to dressle
ere no feeling when we are together WHY DOES IT
NOT ONE TALK TO ME WHY

ME ASLEEP OR AWAKE.

GOTE ME HELDLEY SECTIONED whNT
IS MY LIVE A LIE.
E THE CURRENT RELATIONSHIP SHAT.
need someone to untidy.

ed to be with me.
EXPALANDED

51

While I had the pneumonia, my mouth would constantly fill with phlegm from my lungs which I had to spit out into a bowl, eventually a gadget a bit like a turkey baster attached via a tube to a container by the bed was provided which had a vacuum function to suck my mouth out. I assumed the container was hidden away somewhere out of view but apparently not, and my visitors were rewarded with a view of a large glass container full of what looked like wallpaper paste marbled with something black and green. Initially the nurses would do this for me, after a while I was left to do it myself.

Pleased with this as I hallucinated that one particular nurse would do this so roughly, sticking it in and around in my mouth so forcibly I'd gag. When I saw her, I'd use all the strength I had to hold my teeth together as she attempted to poke it through them. This was so real to me, I still remember the sensation of the plastic rubbing on my teeth and gums as a gap though was being sort, and the soreness of my gums. I actually mentioned it to the ward sister. One day as the nursing team, changed to the evening shift, I saw her waking into the ward. I heard her talking to her colleague's behind the ward station "That's him." I was still effectively fixed to the bed by the various lines attached to me. With trepidation I contemplated on what this night would have in store for me. Continuing with the theme of the best form of defence being attack I decided to tackle this head on and asked for the nurse to sit with me for a chat. I attempted to apologise and explain why this misunderstanding had happened, I'm absolutely sure it wasn't intended, I was just too weak to communicate to her that it was uncomfortable.

The poor woman just had this look I can only describe as a combination of, "what the... is going on? disbelief, horror, hurt, shock and what is this loony talking about?" She composed herself and asked if it was another nurse in the shift that looked like her, I'm guessing she was also from the Far East.

"I'm really very sorry it must have been her," she walked off and asked her to sit with me – the same conversation, same reaction. *Well done Pete*, I'd manage to horribly insult two wonderful caring people in the space of 15 minutes, not my proudest moment, if of course they actually existed at all. Unfortunately, I was still away with the fairies and still considered that they may be very accomplished actors. Again, with hindsight, this was one of those very confusing occasions where the room looked normal but my mind could make up events so convincingly that my memory of it is indistinguishable from those of events that actually did happen. Needless to say, the evening passed without incident.

I seem to remember the strong medication required to beat off the meningitis was a two-week course that had now come to an end, so I was on fewer drugs and the number of lines into both wrists slowly reduced, which made everything easier. As with a NG feeding tube in my nose, a catheter elsewhere, cannulas in both wrists, tapped tubes in and out, one for taking blood out regularly and one for medication in, I couldn't move much. As I couldn't swallow all medication had to be administered intravenously, even paracetamol which was mixed in water and squirted into one of the wrist cannula's with a syringe, accompanied with that strange warming sensation shooting up the inside of my forearm. Turning in bed was awkward or impossible as all the lines would tangle up. This was really unnatural for me as I'm a natural fidget sleeper. Getting out of bed to sit in the bedside chair was time consuming task and required a nurse to sort out the lines and help me into the chair and then sort the lines out again, easily 10 to 15 minutes and the same in reverse to get me back into bed. Initially I'd only be in the chair for half an hour or so, but you have to start somewhere.

Chapter Five

On the general ward

29 February (Monday)

You are transferred to Creaton Ward. You are less confused and your condition is more stable.

Only Trish, George, Kate, David and Hazel had been in to see me up till then, I couldn't cope with anyone else. On the general ward I started to see other family members and then friends from my village.

I didn't record the day the catheter finally came out, but it was about this time. I had big concerns about this as I had no sensation of urinating at all. As I had lost so much sensation down the whole right side of my body, I was worried that this was permanent and that I would be incontinent. I was very relieved, literally, that everything was fine.

At about this time, having survived, the focus changed to getting back to doing things that were second nature only a short time ago. It's particularly shocking how much can be lost in such a short time, things feel so unnatural and awkward even being upright in a chair, let alone walking around, it all made me feel dizzy and nauseous. It took some time to move on from the feeling of *this will never feel natural again* and to build some confidence. The muscles in my arms and legs virtually disappeared and barely seamed to create a bump under the bed sheets. Decades of being reasonably strong, fit and healthy all but wiped out in just two weeks by an incy wincy little bug.

1 March (Tuesday)

Looking back through the notes, including A&E, I was actually moved 10 times back and forth through the various wards, which considering the mental state I was in was quite unsettling. Add this to the number of times I hallucinated a move to some pretty bizarre places by some pretty bizarre methods, it was all pretty confusing. I was very relieved to be told during my third week, now in Creation Ward, that I'd be here until I was to be discharged. However, a while later Nurse S1 told me she'd had had a request to have me moved again to another ward as this ward was generally for patients even less independent than even I'd become. She had said no, because the whole team here had seen the state of me when I arrived, and they all wanted to be there and watch me eventually walk out. I was very relieved, and deeply moved by the sentiment.

2 March (Wednesday)

I noted that Wednesdays were my critical weighting days. I was transferred to a wheelchair with built-in scales, 64kg a little over 10 stone, not sure about the accuracy of this. This was my first time out of bed and I was rather slumped in the wheelchair like a partially deflated balloon.

3 March (Thursday)

The double vision that started on the 22 February was much improved. I woke up and looked at the clock on the wall opposite, it was round again instead of the horizontal figure of eight that I was becoming used to. I noted that I could now almost shut my left eye and was also able to read much easier.

A trip to the X-ray department was planned for a video fluoroscopy to be done to assess my swallow reflex. This is a continuous X-ray image on a monitor, much like an X-ray movie. I was in a wheelchair and had to hold the trace fluid in my mouth, and then swallow when I was told to, not very successfully as not much was working and I'd forgotten how to force it.

The next time you're sitting in the waiting area at the X-ray department for an hour with several other people for the appointment you had booked two months earlier and a porter arrives with someone who is seen immediately and you hide your slight annoyance but understand… that was once me… sorry.

After almost three weeks in bed the physio got me standing up for the first time and helped me up to a

Zimmer frame. My feet didn't leave the ground but with help I shuffled the equivalent of around six paces, with Trish pushing the two-wheeled stands that were holding my feeding bag and saline drip along behind. I'll never forget the look of horror on my sister-in-law Sue's, face. It was either the first or second time she has seen me since I'd become ill, I expect the change in me from three weeks or so earlier was rather extreme. I slowly turned around shuffled back and collapsed onto the bed exhausted.

4 March (Friday)

After yesterday's first walk, I was encouraged to push myself to do more, I had regular visits from the physio who would get me out of bed and walking with the Zimmer frame. I was taken in a wheelchair to the gym for the first and last time in my life, funny never really pictured myself in a gym, especially attempting a five-step staircase. The session went pretty well so the physio took me off the oxygen that I'd been on since 23 February. I could finally ditch the irritating tube with the projections up my nostrils. I had been on the lowest setting of 1 litre flow per minute for a while, around 24 per cent oxygen which is only a little above what would be available naturally. I was determined to walk back to the wards but had to admit defeat and completed the journey in the wheelchair.

My first solo destination with the Zimmer frame was the toilet, around 10 metres way, then eventually the length of the ward corridor. I have forgotten how many paces that was, but that number gave me a target, then to build up the number of corridor lengths. Then start on the short distance on crutches and gradually build up the distance, then a walking stick, then try it without having to stare at the floor, then finally unsupported.

It was as a result of one of these early corridor walks I discovered the whereabouts of patient X, the very trying individual who was constantly demanding the nurses to do something for him "NOW", he asked them to bring clothing or attend to something in a raised voice. He was generally loud and disruptive early in the morning and late in the evening and, I have to say very unappreciative of his wife who had to bus in every visiting time and bring in whatever he'd demanded the previous day. He looked rather older than I'd imagined from his strong booming voice, as he sat in his bedside chair, dressed, serenely asleep, yes daytime and asleep, how dare he appear so oblivious to the chaos he created around him while he was awake? If I had actually had the strength to kick out from my Zimmer or bend down and shout in his ear to wake him, I would have done.

5 and 6 March

Rather bizarrely around this time, I had constant hiccups which lasted for around three days, this made going to sleep a little difficult. I couldn't just relax into a sleep but had to wait until I got so tired, I just dropped off. I'd wake up without hiccups and think, *Okay great,* then after about 5 to10 seconds later it would start again. Also, my diaphragm would just seem to lock up after an intake of breath, no warning, a normal breath in then nothing for a few seconds which was a bit alarming.

7 March (Monday)

The physio was surprised and very pleased with my progress today.

On the general ward, I steadily got stronger and I remember seeing a guy visit the ward outside of the normal visiting hours, clearly a very grateful former patient eagerly returning to thank the nurses who had given him so much care. Lovely to see, but as an outsider to this relationship the way the dynamics had fundamentally changed was very informative. Before, he was the unwell patient being well looked after by caring nurses, and now he was an appreciative visitor wishing to pass on his joy and thanks to busy working nurses, happy to see him but massively under pressure to deliver equal care to the next person. On reflection it was yet further confirmation of what I'd witnessed all the time really. It's way more than a job, the nurses really do genuinely care for you, and if you're in a bed you are the most important person to them. But when you walk out, they have to move on, how can anyone carry that amount of cumulative baggage? I made my first considered absolute decision in a long time, real progress indeed. Note to self: when my day comes, before I walk out of the general ward, hug everyone, thank them and don't come back.

8 March (Tuesday)

I noted that everything sounded louder. Particularly when there were groups of people, individual sounds sometimes seemed to merge into one uncomfortable wall of noise. A second trip to the X-ray department was planned for a further video fluoroscopy to be done to assess my swallow reflex.

9th March (Wednesday)

Wednesday, critical weighting day. I transferred to the wheelchair with the built-in scales, 71kg a little over 11 stone.

As my situation and prospects improved, what was important changed. On admission to ICU keeping me clean was way down the agenda, after a few days I stunk, apparently, so I've been told.

Initially I wasn't really thinking about this or pretty much anything else actually. As it looked more likely I'd survive, I was bed washed each morning by the nurses. As I got a little stronger on the general ward, I gradually took over more of this myself. The morning routine slowly evolved into the curtains drawn, being presented with a washing bowl of warm soapy water, a heap of wet wipes and clean pyjamas and then after that the bed linen was changed. When I did start to actively address hygiene and appearance, I remember, after being washed one morning sitting up in the bed and looking at my hands and feeling my unkempt beard and thinking *which job should I tackle today, cut my finger nails or trim my beard?*

10 March (Thursday)

I had a visit from SALT they showed me some further jaw exercises to work on improving my jaw opening. I was restricted in how much I was able to open my jaw, at a very tight squeeze I could just about manage two fingers between my front teeth if I cheated a bit. That's also not wide enough to brush your back teeth very well. I was allowed a beaker of water to practise sipping and swallowing and was told no more than two or three sips at a time. A bit messy for a while. That night I couldn't sleep and decided to pass time by doing some water sipping exercises, it went surprisingly well so I did some more, by the time SALT came to see me in the morning I'd finished the ¾ litre jug of water I'd been left with, much to their surprise. This luckily laid the foundations for the prospect of being discharged with a liquid diet rather than the planned Percutaneous Endoscopic Gastrostomy (PEG) fitted to my stomach, this was a tube which passed through my skin into my stomach, which would be used to feed me. This would replace the NG feeding tube in my nose as I couldn't be discharged with this feeding method.

11 March (Friday)

Earlier I had no interest or energy to do anything, even though Trish had bought me a radio in to listen to as well as magazines and newspapers to read, they all remained piled up, unused. Today I asked Trish to bring an old smart phone in so I could keep in touch, Kate got rid of all the old stuff on it and charged it up. I sent my first text to Trish.

I had my third trip to the X-ray department for a further video fluoroscopy, went pretty well today, I'm now allowed limited drinks, hot, chilled or sparkling – first cup of tea.

I wanted to try some solid food this weekend, I'd developed my first food craving, breakfast, bowl of Rice Krispies with chilled fresh milk, don't know why I never have them at home. This was as a result of being encouraged by Nurse H, he would tempt me to try things, I was never quite sure if this was "official" and under the advice the dietitian or him independently willing me on, pushing me to progress. As my swallow was still very poor, I was concerned about letting something into my lungs and causing another infection.

I next saw him after the in-house magazine interview 2 November 2016 which took place in the seminar room in ICU. When we finished the interview, some pictures were taken within the Unit, by then he'd moved from

Creaton Ward to become an ICU nurse. We managed a hug and a catch-up chat.

Most nights on the general ward there seemed to be someone struggling and in some form of distress, either feeling ill, missing their spouse/family or generally being disruptive, shouting unreasonably for the nurses attention, or just softly, painfully chanting the names of loved ones relentlessly for hours. This was a little annoying and made relaxing difficult, you had to work hard at not hearing it, mind you there were probably some evenings that was me. One night there was patient a couple of bays away from mine, who was clearly having the most awful time, sobbing and distressed. There was this young Caribbean nurse that was sitting and talking with him for ages, comforting him. I'll never forget the sound of her voice, so calming like slow flowing melting chocolate with that lovely hint of a relaxed Jamaican accent. Eventually she talked him down, she just wouldn't give up on him, he didn't stand a chance. Her voice just drifted through the dimly lit, otherwise quiet ward and hugged you. I'm reminded of that every time I hear that accent.

I do wonder what became of the five other patients who I shared the bay of six beds with at the end, my bed was halfway down the left side of the bay. The charming guy that was to my right, next to the corridor, who when I was feeling a little stronger would have short chats with now again. The guy to my left, next to the window, had lost the sight in one eye and was facing the loss of the other and very calmly and eloquently explained to his consultant, that having carefully considered everything, having had a full active life, wonderful long marriage, lovely grandchildren, great holidays, could not face his future blind. Unless they could guarantee to preserve the sight in his remaining eye, he had decided that he would respectfully and without fuss decline food and medicine. The new person opposite to the left, next to the window, who wasn't there long enough for me to know anything about. The chap directly opposite me who apparently had a major open wound that wouldn't heal and was under constant pain management and clearly subdued and quiet with the medication he was on. The guy opposite to me to the right, next to the corridor, who among other issues had some sort of dementia, and was convinced I was Dave. This was not constantly or all day but now and again he would get very frustrated and shout in angry disbelieve that Dave wouldn't interact with him and continually ignored him.

12 March (Saturday)

No contest, best day in quite a while. As yesterday video fluoroscopy went so well, I took my pill medication orally for the first time. Also, Kate put some credit on the TV so I could watch England play Wales in the Six Nations rugby, great game, 25-21 win.

I had my first trip out of the ward that didn't involve a porter taking me to another ward or department. Trish took me out in a wheelchair. This was a very welcome pleasure, a bit of a holiday away from the ordeal, slightly marred by the guy opposite (Dave's mate) pointing at me and accusing me, in a raised voice, of nicking his stuff. I wasn't going to allow him to spoil my day, so we made our getaway anyway. We toured the hospital corridors and then went out to the car park for my first feel of the outside, away from everyone else. It felt a bit like a first date, just Trish and me, the breeze on my face, so refreshing. Then we stopped off at the café for a cup of tea on our way back to the ward and met up with Dave and Hazel.

Generally, on the ward, I tried to avoid eye contact with Dave's mate as much as possible as this seemed to encourage him to attempt to talk to his old friend, I wasn't sure how to handle this. I did have to remind myself that I was a patient as well, I really didn't need this or actually have any spare energy to console him and didn't even know how to. The nurses did their best to attempt this. It did eventually kick off. "Dave, Dave, Dave, DAVE," he shouted at me with visible anger in his contorted face.

I sat up in bed and pointed at him "MY NAME IS PETE. DO YOU HEAR ME? PETE. I'LL TALK TO YOU IF YOU USE MY NAME, I'M PETE." Then I fell back into the pillow with my hands over my face. Several nurses appeared to calm probably the lamest altercation between two guys that there has ever been and which was already finished. Shortly afterwards he was swapped with an empty bed which saw a stream of transient patients spending a short time there until I was discharged. This targeted assertion of my name unfortunately missed by one bed, as the wife of the subdued chap with the wound opposite me explained to Trish at one of the visiting times, she was really surprised that her husband actually knew my name.

Now having got the phone yesterday, during the night with the boredom of again not being able to sleep very well and with nothing to do, I made the mistake of googling bacterial meningitis, what big mistake that was, just stopped myself short of having to push the call button to request a bed pan. Why is it you seldom google anything that's going well with your health, only problems and then naturally gravitate to the worst scenario? Although I have to say that on this occasion, as scary as what I was reading was, the reality was far worse.

13 March (Sunday)

An exciting day, I had my first shower in a month. I was allowed to sit on a plastic patio chair in the shower as long as I didn't put my head under the water to wash my hair. I was not allowed to do this while my feed tube (NG) was still in place. As this ward was generally for patients less mobile than even I'd become, I noticed the one available shower didn't get used, that was my incentive to crack on.

At last some semblance of a return to normality, I got up when the trolley full of fresh pyjamas arrived, then I picked a pair out with a fresh towel. There wasn't a queue for the shower, so it was mine. I took ages in there as it was still a really exhausting effort. By the time I got back to my bed it had been made with clean linen. And I got plugged into my feeding bag.

Trish took me out and about for another walk in the wheelchair, just the two of us, another great day.

14 March (Monday)

I had another visit from SALT this morning they say that I'm handling fluids so well now, that the NG feeding tube should be able to come out permanently today.

Also, I spoke to the dietitian, in light of recent developments she was now working on preparing a fluid diet ready for my discharge. Things seem to be progressing fast now.

I messaged Trish, George and Kate, 21.18pm, NG out, finally nothing attaching me to anything, I have the freedom to fidget around as much as I like. I can also lie down in bed completely flat for the first time rather than be propped up to allow the NG feeding to work by gravity. I'll be able to get fully under the shower in the morning.

15th March (Tuesday)

Reality check this morning; I was a bit too ambitious. Having been encouraged to finally to try my bowl of

Rice Krispies with chilled milk for breakfast, unfortunately I struggled so much swallowing I had to give up, having coughed some up from my lungs. This was sort of a good sign, as it showed my cough reflex was strong enough to clear my lungs if I had to.

I was Nil by Mouth for approximately four weeks. I'd been allowed limited drinks for around 4 days now but this evening I had my one and only hospital meal, tomato and basil soup, a small pot of jelly and another of ice cream, the first tastes in my mouth for a month. On the general ward, three times a day I had watched and smelt three course meals arrive for, and be consumed by everyone else. While a bag full of murky pond water hanging above me took a couple of hours to disappear up my nose two or three times a day.

The meals were delivered by the wonderful ward domestic, Mrs L, she did a fantastic job delivering food, drinks and cleaning the ward. She did tell me that it upset her to walk past me all the time delivering food to everyone else and suggested tomorrow trying cornflakes soaked in slightly warmer milk, only leaving them for a while, as this worked for her old dog that didn't have any teeth.

The combination of the difficulty I had in swallowing, together with the restriction I had in how much I could open my jaw, was an issue long after I was discharged. To eat an apple, I'd have to stab it Dracula style with my top teeth and rip a chunk out chew it forever and sip water to swallow it. This was very frustrating as I've always been a big eater of all fresh fruit, right from my days as a youngster scrumping off the village allotments and orchards. The swallowing very gradually improved in stages, nothing changed for months then there was an improvement, then it plateaued for months and so on. I managed to very slowly eat my first normal lunchtime sandwich without sipping water after 18 months. Generally, I have wraps instead of sliced bread now.

SALT said they would be happy for me to go home, they're writing up their notes to discharge me form their care. Had my fourth trip to the X-ray department for a further video fluoroscopy to be done, monitoring how my swallow reflex was developing.

16 March (Wednesday)

To my mind a momentum for me to be discharged and the excitement built from Monday, the physio had discharged me from his care, in the light of me finally being able to swallow water and my dietitian coming up with a suitable liquid diet, SALT with a few conditions were happy to discharge me from their care. All lines were out of me. Today, the D word, discharge from the hospital was mentioned again. I was elated, it felt realistic. I thought of the decision I'd made a few days earlier about goodbyes. Don't know what I did when I was insane but when I was me, I never called out for the nurses I always pressed the button and waited. However, this time the truly amazing Nurse T was as usual rushing past to attend to something and I called out her name, she stopped turned around and walked up to me and asked what's wrong. I was sitting in the bedside chair with my hand on the tray trolley which was across my lap, "It looks as though I'm going to be discharged this afternoon," I said. She put both her hands on both of mine.

"If I don't get the opportunity to say it then, I want to say it now – thank you," I said.

She let go of my hands and put her arms around my neck we hugged and she said, "I was here and saw you the day you came in. It's been so lovely watching you get better day by day." We both had tears for a few seconds, she then carried on being absolutely amazing. On reflection, it sounds implausible, but up until that moment, I hadn't fully connected the not surviving bit with not going home again. This was the first time I'd really allowed myself to consider that this ordeal was actually coming to an end, there was something afterwards, I would go home. I can't remember before having the right words, at the right time, one of greatest moments of my life. Flushed with this success when I was finally discharged, I tracked everyone down on the ward that I recognised hugged them and said thank you. Trish did explain to me sometime after that I may have committed a major faux pas with Nurse L, who was a lady of the Muslim faith and unfortunately she didn't escape the hug, such a caring person, with the most deft technique with a difficult NG tube and tips like using lemon juice to help with the nausea. On reflection, I do hope I didn't cause offence with a spontaneous genuine act of gratitude.

As the usual Wednesday morning's round by the consultant approached, I was so looking forward to seeing him. Unfortunately, he didn't appear, however two more junior colleagues did, we spoke briefly and finally one of them said they'd try and get the discharge hopefully for the weekend, that was maybe two or three more days and nights.

"No, you don't understand? I can't be here another night," I said.

"Maybe Thursday or Friday then," they said and off they went. I couldn't remember the last time I had had tears in my eyes and this was the second time in a couple of hours. Nurse S2 walked past and I was greeted with the usual, "Alright darling how you doing?"

"Well up until around 20 minutes ago fine," I said.

She came to my bedside and with a concerned face, "Why what's happened?"

The right time for anything is when it feels right and it felt right for me now. I knew that without the treatment and care from the whole team I'd be dead, or have bits missing, they had now done all they possibly could to bring me to this point, but could add nothing more. I needed to go home, be with my family and friends and start my recovery. Just bed blocking here was achieving nothing, if anything it was now holding me back. "I can't do another night here; I'm thinking I should self-discharge," I said.

"You leave this to me," she said and off she went. Nothing to do with this I'm sure, but within a couple of hours or so the consultant and his entourage were at my bedside. After a few questions, I was okayed to go.

I rang Trish immediately, "When you come in this afternoon, bring some clothes please, I'm coming home."

So, other than the obvious one, no regrets and only one thing left unsaid which is not bad considering. Twice in the last week of general ward, the individual curtains were drawn around each of us, once in the bay of six beds that I was in. This particular time I could glimpse though a gap in the curtains at the passage of the large black zipped bag on a gurney stretcher trolley going past. The curtains were then pulled back to reveal a nurse making up an empty bed with new linen, having first changed the mattress. My bed was halfway down the left side of the bay, a chap diagonally opposite me to the left, next to the window had passed away. I'd heard he was in his nineties. He'd arrived a few days earlier and every visiting time at least two generations of his family came to see him, the youngsters were well behaved, they all stopped as long as they could and kissed him as they left. I never heard him call out in pain or distress, even though the lonely nights. The nurses were attentive, talking to him as often as they were able to and helping him to eat and regularly drink. They treated him with a charming respect and dignity. All in all, it seemed to me, that this brief period was a good end to a clearly treasured long life, spent well. I think it was his granddaughter who came in to collect some of his belongings from the bedside; I watched her as she walked out past the foot of my bed. I really wanted to tell her all this, but somehow, I just couldn't and the moment just slipped away. I was reminded of thoughts I'd had at a couple of key moments where I'd considered that if what I was experiencing right then, were my last moments, my last thoughts, they would never be known to those closest to me. The poignancy of the moment would be lost and could only be condensed into a single sentence of lifeless text starting something like, "Unfortunately Mr Smith didn't…" Generally I'll be very much better prepared next time.

Chapter Six

After discharge

During the first year of recovery I also, rather shockingly, discovered what an absolute dinosaur I am. Spread out over the year I had several visits back to NGH. Each time, in preparation, I'd polish my shoes put a good shirt and jacket on and get to the hospital early, I just couldn't help myself. Silly really, I wanted to show the "hospital" that I valued what was done for me, that all the effort and resources lavished on me were worthwhile and I intended to make the good use of this extra time. For me this didn't mean seeing the rest of the world or running a marathon, the most important things require very little travelling and virtually no physical effort, it's the little things, the everyday details and people that are the most important to me.

I had follow-up chats with ICU follow-up nurse Emma Madden at two months, six months and a year after my discharge. As an outpatient, I had meetings to check on progress with SALT and Nutrition and Dietetics on 21 March and the 20 June. A return to the X-ray department, 23 June for another video fluoroscopy to check how my swallow reflex was developing. It's interesting the boost and the great value even the smallest amount of personal human contact can give you to lift your spirits, on returning to the X-ray department, I was greeted by the charming Radiographer L.

"Oh Hi Peter, nice to see you again… looking good… right you know the routine stand there… Ooh nice shirt, don't want to mess that up, should maybe take it off if you don't mind."

There was a follow-up check CT scan of my head on the 4 July, and a meeting with the neurologist on the 19 August. I also had the first of two consultations with wellbeing psychologist on the 12 September.

My bloods were taken and over 30 tests done, for diabetes, thyroid function and all manner of other organ functions, more than 10 on my heart alone. All fell within a normal range, which considering the sustained beating I'd taken, I was very pleased about. I really didn't want to have to be reliant on long-term medication for the first time in my life, it was very important to me to have as little permanent damage as possible.

6 May 2016: First ICU follow-up meeting.

At the end of my two months after discharge meeting with Nurse Emma, she offered me a tour of the ICU, which I was very comfortable to take her up on. What a weird sensation that was. I didn't recognise any of it at all. I didn't go into the room with the single bed, not that I had a problem with that, but it just didn't happen, too much to take in. Being greeted by so many smiling faces clearly so happy to see me again – and looking rather better than the last time they'd seen me. But I didn't recognise anyone. Seeing such poorly patients also really rammed home the fact that had been me just a short while ago and how well I was doing. HDU looked very familiar, I could identify the bed I was in and recognised the view from the window. Although an image kept popping up in my head of my bed being central in small circular room like a castle turret with windows all around that flooded the room with bright daylight. No sign of the "Thunderbirds" ramp that was gone, don't know how they'd managed to hide that.

Critical care is a uniquely unusually environment, everything, every day is life and death, extremes of emotions. All emotions are heightened just having passed through this environment of ICU and HDU. Days of all-consuming worry, great relief or total tragedy, with only timeless waiting in between. Even with the memories so fresh in my mind, I didn't feel hesitant about returning, quite the reverse in fact, this was the place, that ultimately produced a very positive outcome for me. I felt very comfortable, at home there. I felt humbled to have had all this massive resource and so many skilled professionals focused on the survival of little ole me. There's a strange juxtaposition of being glad to be out but almost missing being there in hospital, wanting to be there until I actually felt completely better, as I used to be. Maybe I just like being pampered.

7 October 2016. My second ICU follow-up meeting, six months after discharge.

By now the three-month holiday period after discharge was well and truly over and the long grind of recovery was underway. I began to be more aware of issues, my mind had now chosen to begin to process all that had happened. I started to have problems with sleeping and anxiety. It was very reassuring to discuss these with Emma, she could either explain what was going on to me, make suggestions and where appropriate and necessary, was very prompt in writing to my GP to suggest referrals where there were concerns.

Having got out, away from the dedicated 24/7 care of professionals a door slams shut and you're on your own. After a while there was very much a feeling of abandonment; although I was technically "cured" I really didn't physically feel very much better. Wounds that can't be seen or measured are so slow to heal. I was also made aware of the work Nurse Emma does with a group called ICU Steps who have groups all over the country. It's essentially a relaxed, informal support group for ex-ICU patients and relatives. It has to be run by a current clinician, usually an ICU nurse. Its run entirely by volunteers and receives no funding other than donations, all money raised goes straight to supporting patient and relatives.

10 February 2017. My third and last ICU follow-up meeting, a year after discharge.

Emma greeted me with congratulations, as at that point, I was officially recorded in the hospital statistics as having survived, which is the normal routine for patients who pass through the Unit.

It was at about this time I went to my first ICU Steps meeting. Having been a self-employed homeworker for almost 30 years I'm hardwired to work alone and was unsure if I'd get anything out of this. I decided to go along anyway, no harm in trying.

The meetings are around every six weeks for a couple of hours with soft, hot and cold drinks and biscuits. Sometimes we talk about our experiences, sometimes not. But having the opportunity to talk with others and have this amount of access to an active ICU nurse is incredible, much better than 10 to15 minutes with a GP, what a luxury.

I've met a group of amazing people with a variety of shared experiences that I have an instant bond with, an instinctive understanding and empathy with. An exclusive club, the rest of you are muggles. A group with whom I can talk openly to, if I want to, without boring them. Getting your story out of you is the key to recovering, the more you talk the more normal it feels and the more accepting of it you become. A strange transition occurs, slides over you, sharing small successes.

When someone there says I know what you mean/how you felt, you know they actually do and your experiences were not unique. As you progress you see the importance of this and you want to convey that to those who are just starting. One thing is sure, there will be others to follow.

A relatively common theme for hallucinating seems to be water related – swimming, floating, sailing, oceans etc. Mine was on a very large catamaran yacht with most of my family and a particular nurse who I remembered, she was my personal medic on the yacht. This must have been while I had the oxygen nasal cannula in place as she was constantly nagging me about this. Although all my memories of this time were of having a tunnel view, no peripheral vision, a circular image of what was immediately in front of me with a black area around it. It's believed that the water theme may due to the Alternating Pressure Air Mattresses that are used to that help prevent bed sores. Air is pumped into different chambers of the mattress to move the pressure points around, so you get this constant slow undulating movement of the mattress.

Chapter Seven

Recovery

I got home slept well and exercised regularly, slowly built up my strength, and was back to normal after nine or ten months, with a few hiccups along the way. Well that was plan A. However, unfortunately I had to initiate plan B, C, D and E.

I just felt – empty, there is no other way of describing it really. Trish did say that I felt fragile to hug, as though she could break me in two, which she found very upsetting.

The first night at home in bed was heaven, the best ever, bar none, completely dark and quiet. The first few days or so were experimental, trying out various foods to see what I could swallow, so I did not have to rely on the prescription of 90 200ml bottles of Fortisip which I took home. Fortisip is a heavily fortified milkshake-based drink each containing 320 calories, so six pretty much give you enough of everything to sustain you through the day. The idea being to eat as normally as possible and use the Fortisip to top up as required.

The first three months after discharge were the holiday period. I slept well and started daily short walks around the village and gradually built this up to a mile-long circular route, which after a while I did two or three times a day. I gradually became more aware of things that were wrong. It wasn't because I was getting any worse, just waking up. As I began to get even a little stronger and attempted returning to a normal live, the mist started to lift and the new me slowly began to emerge.

Having lost almost 20 per cent of my body weight, mostly of muscle, everything was hard work. It was a long process adding weight and pushing myself to exercising enough to turn this into muscle. Trish would cook as usual and have what she wanted, then I'd have to add all the normal bad things, loads of butter, cream etc and finish with an afters, full fat yogurt with dried or fresh fruit and honey, trifles, cheesecake, all much easier to swallow and loaded with calories.

Building strength took time but went rather well I thought, building up stamina was a completely different issue, it has taken so much longer. I had no reserves of strength to draw on and no warning when it was coming to an end. When it was all used up, it was gone instantly and I'd feel awful, lightheaded, nauseous, wobbly and would have to sit down. I'd be on the verge of tears of frustration at this imposition of this new limit on what I was now physically capable of. I suppose this happens gradually to everyone as you age over a long period but having to make all this adjustment instantly is difficult. Initially when I reached this stage, I didn't recover that day. After a year or so passed I got better at recognising when I was doing too much, as I got stronger if I'd sit down for an hour or so I would recover and feel better, although I wouldn't continue working. As the muscles all over my body started to get a little stronger, those in my right arm didn't. I'm right-handed but my left arm soon became the stronger. I'm still much less able to do physical work than I was. If I do even moderate manual work, I always get an uncomfortable pins and needles in my right arm, and an aching feeling a bit like hot air blasting longways through my bones. A couple of ibuprofen tablets normally help with this.

I generally had very poor balance, I couldn't walk in a straight line, looking either way up the road before I crossed made me a little nauseous and wobbly. The numbness from the top of my head to my toes down the right side of my body hasn't changed, everything feels at room temperature. A thousand times I must have, as feels natural, turned on a kitchen or bathroom tap with my left hand and held a finger of my right hand under the water to test the temperature, only to discover I can't feel anything and have to swap over. Or have picked cutlery out of the recently finished dishwasher and put it away with my right hand and have to drop it if I used my left hand. I burnt my hand getting something out of the oven and barely noticed until I got the smell. Pain generally on the whole right side of my body is no longer the instant instinctive fast defensive pull way, but a slow build-up of an uncomfortable pins and needles which leaves plenty of time to acquire damage. I once got my finger shut in a doorway, the nail turned all black and eventually fell off without any discomfort.

I look in the mirror and see my uneven eyebrows, the stationary left one and slightly dropped left corner of my mouth. These get more pronounced as I get tired and my left eye narrows. Sometimes my mouth can't keep up with my brain and I stumble over words or mumble incoherently. Every time I smile or laugh it feels as though I've got a strip of surgical support tape stuck from my temple to my jaw, as muscles on this left side of my face either don't move at all or not enough and they work against each other.

The airways connecting my ears, nose and throat sometimes completely block and my voice sounds nasally like with a bad cold, and I have to breathe through my mouth. When this happens, which is for a period every day, or occasionally most of the day, I can't talk and breathe, or eat and breathe at the same time. So, doing either means I'm holding my breath and have to catch one wherever I can, or take a deeper breath to compensate every now and then, which is very frustrating and can actually be quite tiring. A functioning nose is a really good idea, who thought of that. I need to sip water with a lot of what I eat even now, so items that started warm on the plate go down stone cold. This has improved, initially I'd sip water with everything remotely solid, lumps of red meat are just not an option at all. Initially not much tasted of anything, this has improved a little but all wine still tastes like the same strong vinegar. I'm generally the last at the table to finish eating and need not to talk to limit this as much as possible, social dinning is not quite the pleasure it once was.

I didn't drink any alcohol for well over a year probably nearer two. Not that I was advised not to, but for all that time I never really felt that well, it's best described as how you feel the day after you've drunk too much alcohol the night before, the next day you're able do everything you want to, but are looking forward to tomorrow because you know you'll be back to normal then, except that tomorrow never arrives. I was also told by ICU follow-up nurse Emma that, after a major illness your body is constantly working on overdrive on repairing itself 24/7. This burns calories and can make you feel tried. I decided not to give my body any additional unnecessary self-inflected work to do, like clearing out alcohol. I was determined to make as full a recovery as possible, whatever it took, for as long as necessary. I was set an artificial recovery date at an appointment I had with the neurologist; he had actually said that after 18 months to two years what I was left with would likely be permanent. I selectively heard what I wanted to hear and took this to mean I'd be recovered in that time. I did have to regroup and have a major rethink just after this time, to adjust to the reality that I'm never going to be as I once was.

In comparison to other people who have lived through what I have, these all seem pretty trivial, I am still here and in one piece. Although every day these issues are unavoidable reminders of that time, and there are more reminders that I've collected over the next four years that have added to them.

Also, it isn't exclusively the severity of the deficits that become problematic, on your down days it's also the longevity of them. Every day, permanent, the rest of your life, it's a long time, you'd eventually get fed up even with your favourite meal after every day for four years.

The process of the holiday period drifting to an end was explained to me as a well-documented progression. When something traumatic happens that you're going to struggle with, as a defence mechanism your brain blanks it out so you can concentrate on getting through it. These events are only stored away for future reference not deleted. When you've sufficiently recovered, all the feelings and emotions, as they should have been at the time, will then resurface and be just as powerfully as they should have been at the time. For me this wasn't so much debilitating traumatic flash backs, more vivid memories and crushing anxiety.

This gradually became a sleeping issue. It started with a general nonspecific anxiety that built slowly as the evening progressed and I became increasingly nervous, very uncomfortable with the thought of sleeping. When

I'd get into bed as soon as my head touched the pillow the hit of adrenaline was like a simultaneous punch to the stomach and slap around my face. I'd be wide awake and compelled to get up with a powerful fight and flight response. I'd be on a big high for around an hour or so. This would happen several times a night, no matter how tired I was, and I wouldn't get any sleep at all. The next day would pass as a sort of zombie-like blur. My fear of sleeping was so powerfully, my sub-conscious mind wouldn't allow me to nap during the day. I would just wait for the evening to arrive, hoping that my basic human need to sleep would be stronger than the escalating anxiety as night fell. There was also an urgency to fill each day with things to do, ideally a number of different things to make the day seem longer. I couldn't stop myself thinking that doing nothing was wasting valuable time, sleeping is unproductive, a finite amount of sand slipping through my fingers never to be replaced.

This all worsened and would build-up in the early evening. Typically, I'd be relaxing and watching television with Trish and it would start. The restlessness would build into an awful feeling of anxiety. I'd then pace around the house and no matter how hard I consciously tried to relax and think positive thoughts, *I'm alive and well, things are going great, I'm really lucky,* everything all counted for nothing. I'd feel emotional and on the verge of tears. I couldn't sit still and had to be on the move, the thought of all this then started the doubt as to whether I'd manage to get to sleep later or not. This anxiety would add to the crushing pressure I felt, and the situation would spiral out of control. Time seemed to pass more quickly and accelerate to the usual bedtime for everyone else, leaving me floundering on my own, not that having anyone else there would have helped. I needed to be alone to concentrate on trying not to work, at trying to relax. I needed to be sitting down for comfort but wanting to move so I didn't get bored. Driving ticked all the boxes and gave me something else to think about, keeping me in the moment so I've been told. This helped, so inevitably evolved into longer and longer drives. Over time I developed a total circumnavigation of Northampton town avoiding main roads as much as possible, and quietly passing though the lovely countryside and villages. I varied the route a little but this was about 40 to 45-mile round trip, taking between an hour and a quarter and an hour and a half. It started with occasional trip in summer of 2016, it escalated to almost every evening by the summer of 2017, until I was finally done with this by the autumn of 2018. This added around 12,500 extra miles to our car's usual travel, roughly 300 trips over a two to two-and-a-quarter year period.

At my worst the evenings and nights became very busy, after dinner I would go for my drive, then spend time some time at home. I'd have my first walk at about 11:30pm and live with whatever happened after that. I did have to become very aware and listen to what my body was communicating. To do whatever I felt was required for as long as was needed. But be alert to whenever I'd finished getting what I need from it, and necessity had turned to habit. Then somehow, I had to develop the strength to stop.

In between failed attempts to sleep at night, I'd take some clothes downstairs and get dressed hoping not to wake Trish, then walk my route around the village again to use up the energy high. This might happen at say around 1.30am, then 3am, 5am and then at 7am I might put the computer on and try and do some work. Sometimes at say anywhere between 3am and 5am, part way around one of my walks, the energy high would disappear and I'd find myself staggering along the road literally fighting to stop myself falling asleep walking, desperately trying to get home before I fell over. I'd fall into bed and shortly after the adrenaline would hit again and my eyes would be wide open. Generally, on alternate nights, 48 hours without sleep, I'd just crash out. I'd wake up and instantly the anxiety would compel me to get out of bed to prevent me from just lying there relaxing in hope of falling asleep again.

Being away from my familiar comfort place, home, exacerbates the sleeping issue, I still haven't slept without Trish. If she hadn't been with me and/or acted as she did on that evening, I clearly would not have survived. This has made taking a holiday, evenings away, even visiting our son in Liverpool rather difficult. Even evenings out became difficult, I'd need to be home by 11pm ish to start my preparations to have any prospect of sleeping. It's also much easier if I've got a normal day, out of bed and working whenever I like. Knowing I have to be out of bed, ready in time to attend a business meeting or book out of accommodation can be the difference between an acceptable sleep and little, or even no sleep at all.

Off-the-shelf sleeping pills, and even Night Nurse, didn't seem to work, they were just not strong enough against the hit when it came. The recommended dose didn't work and just made me feel worse during the next day.

I was prescribed sleeping pills as a temporary measure by my GP, although on researching these later, I decided not to take them as the potential for onerous side effects or comfort seeking accidental long-term addiction, were too bigger price to pay, a short term temporary fix for a long-term issue that may end up in clinical depression, and actually aggravating the insomnia.

Bloods were taken for allergy testing as it was thought the issue with getting blocked up might be an allergic reaction. I had already been messing about with my diet removing dairy products then gluten to no effect. The most likely culprit came out as house dust mites. Although the tests apparently highlight what may be an issue if you were allergic, not if you actually had an allergy. We removed the carpets from the house and installed hard flooring, changed the bed linen and bought the appropriate pillow and mattress covers, got a new HPA filter vacuum cleaner and upped the cleaning routine. I had several months on various prescription antihistamine and steroid nasal spray and tried everything the chemists had, nothing seemed to help. I was referred back to Ear, Nose and Throat (ENT) department at the hospital. The consultant observed I had a deviated septum, a reduced airway through my nose. A septoplasty was required which is a surgical procedure to straighten the bone and cartilage dividing the space between the two nostrils (septum). I also had a reduction of the inferior turbinates. The aim of this procedure (an allergy and sinus treatment) is to shrink swollen nasal turbinates that obstruct the nasal passages. The procedure requires a general anaesthetic. There must be a medical difference between general anaesthetic, sedation and induced coma but my humble civil engineer's brain didn't understand what that was, I've googled it and still don't fully understand. I've got to admit, the whole idea of being in one place, knocked out, moved around, have a medical procedure and then waking up somewhere else, I found totally horrendous. I focused my mind on the prize, if it all went well, I hoped I wouldn't need any medication afterwards, trying to make everything into a positive.

I finally had the operation on 11 October 2017 and after about four days the bleeding finally stopped and eventually the swelling disappeared. Apparently, it will normally take a while to fully appreciate the benefits of this but all the early promise gradually faded away; it made no difference to my situation at all.

On returning to my GP with the same issues she decided to discuss this with the neurologist at the hospital, between them they concluded that I'm more likely to be experiencing "silent migraines", a migraine but thankfully without the excruciating unbearable pain, but dizziness, headaches, weakness and breathing problems etc, with a heightened uncomfortable sensitivity to light and sound.

I tried various migraine drugs with little or no improvement. It seemed that the stronger they got, again the more onerous the potential side effects were and the greater the risk of them become even less effective after long-term use, so a spiralling into taking more and become addicted to the long-term use. This might eventually cause issues with insomnia and clinical depression and would not cure issues but only mask them.

With all options explored and no clear long-term gain in sight I arrived at the only conclusion I felt that I could. That having survived as I had, I had no intention of then medicating myself into future problems, when I'm done with all this, it has to end there.

The solution seemed to be identifying the triggers and avoiding them as much as possible. These, for me are bright lights, daylight of a certain intensity, also bright shop lighting, loud intense sustained sounds that when they reach the level to trigger a reaction seem to merge into an uncomfortable wall of noise. Other triggers seem to be hunger and other things I've not been able to discover yet or this may be as I've said, nonspecific, not relating to anything physical that's happening at the time, which makes avoiding it rather difficult.

With conventional medication exhausted and found not to be effective, for the residual issues only of course, not in the saving of my live. Without conventional medicine and treatment, I would have been dead by 17 February 2016. It was the turn of more unconventional treatments. I couldn't actually say I'd tried everything until I actually had. I tried hypnotherapy, acupuncture and psychotherapy. I read everything I could find, questioned and listened to the various therapist. It's difficult to assess the relative success of these things, nothing is predictable or follows a uniform, linear path there are peaks and troughs. So, assessing the effectiveness of any one thing is very difficult. Eventually I concluded that probably none of these are the magic silver bullet for me, I felt that their strength is in empowering you to heal yourself. The trick is to find the one thing or a combination of things, that does that for you. Maybe I actually needed to try everything, jump through all the hoops, to finally progress to where I am now.

A key moment for me was the first session with the second psychotherapist I saw on 7 August 2018, two and a half years after my illness. It was an hour-long session that overran by at least 20 minutes, in which he took copious notes as I spoke almost continuously. I had used the phase being "frightened to sleep".

On reflection he manipulated the conversation to get me to repeat it, and then immediately interrupted and hit me with his first big punch "But of course you're not are you?" In that split second I felt indignant, he'd begun to lose me. I thought how can you arrive at that after less than an hour, when I'd been living with it all this time. My brain worked in overdrive as I struggled to take this in. His timing was absolutely perfect, like an accomplished stand-up comedian. Then a pause but before I could respond, although he did have my total attention.

"If anything at all, you're frightened of dying while you are asleep, that's a very different issue. You seem to be a reasonably intelligent logical thinking sort of bloke, you were very ill, you're not now. What would you estimate are the chances of you dying in your sleep tonight, tomorrow night, or any at time in the near future actually are – accepting that we will all die at some point in the future?" He left me to stew in this as I fought to keep up, and waited quietly, expectantly for me to respond with something. Eventually "fairly remote" was all I could come up with or think of. He had skilfully shaken me out of my blinkered thinking. I had genuinely thought I'd kept myself flexible, open to new ideas, but on this key issue I hadn't. He'd given my subconscious mind the slap it needed, and the ammunition I required to try a different approach.

I had one other session with him, on 28 August 2018, in which he worked on strengthening my already positive outlook but focusing it much better. Reinforcing the importance of good mental health, wellbeing, all the things that when you're well, you would not consider at all, or dismiss as cliché, tree hugging, and hippy but are actually a very good idea anyway. He convinced me that although my subconscious mind was still trying to protect me from a danger that no longer existed, it wouldn't waste energy on doing this if it could be convinced that it wasn't needed now, and it would eventually give up. But it knows when you're lying, so a battle of attrition had to play out.

It must be said that how I approached this, and how I made sense of it for myself, is all a totally unscientific uncorroborated research study, with a sample population of one.

The conscious and subconscious mind normally work together in a way that just seamlessly deals with everything that you experience. The subconscious mind handling everything that doesn't require a decision: blinking, breathing, smiling when you meet someone you like. If you do something often enough and there are no negative consequences, if you encounter something similar it will make you respond in a similar way automatically. It forms the core of you, the way you are. When something traumatic happens, it protects you from fully experiencing the trauma, in an attempt to help ensure you survive by dealing with it well, being as free from fear as possible.

The conscious mind handles everything else that requires much more effort, it deals with anything you encounter for the first time or that you haven't experienced often enough to be safe to pass over to its buddy. With events that need a decision, it collects information together compares it with anything remotely similar in the database, processes it, and then allows you to activate whatever decision or reaction you've come up with. Medication or an injury to the mind interferes with this happy relationship and can cause a disconnect that can elicit an inappropriate response.

I felt that conventional medication could not alter my inappropriate subconscious response or repair my broken mind. Ultimately the only weapon I have is myself, my mind must repair itself, I must find whatever it is that gives me the ammunition to do this. I don't have to win every battle, there is no point wasting energy on ones that are clearly unwinnable. However, the impossible ones can be rendered irrelevant by eventually winning the war.

I completely changed the way I thought about sleeping, and selflessly threw myself into hobbies and interests that previously I was a little disappointed that I couldn't make very much time for.

I am also pretty fortunate to have a special combination of a strong extended family, and to live in a small caring village environment with good neighbours and great friends. Six of us meet on a Tuesday evening in the local pub and unload whatever has been done to us that week, and between us we put it right. I didn't contribute much for quite a while, I'd sit quietly with my tomato juice with Worcestershire source, enjoying the welcomed break from things, a snapshot reminder of what the undamaged world was like. Even when I didn't particularly feel well enough, I had offers to pick me up and drive me the 200 metres just to get me out and I'd sit there and barely speak all evening. The world is a slightly better place on a Wednesday morning after we'd put it right on a Tuesday night. They'd pop in for a little chat now and again or help me with one of the little projects I'd taken on.

Previously I'd get out of bed, and just couldn't help thinking *how will I sleep tonight?* I was reminded of something I once read somewhere, that if you're struggling with sleep, your preparation for getting ready for a good sleep starts when you get up. I would think, *okay I don't sleep, so what, I'll accommodate this in my day, if I have to put the computer on at 3am and work a bit, well whatever? I'll deal with it and rest when I can. Over the 24 hours I'll do everything I want, but maybe in a weird order at bizarre times. To take the pressure off, I'll try not to think of it as going to bed to sleep, it's lying down for a rest. If I'm not ready to go to sleep, I won't lie there merely reinforcing the connection between lying in bed and not sleeping, I'll get up do something boring until I'm ready. If it's late at night and cold, don't put the heating on or extra clothes, keep it cold. Relish the warmth when you get in bed, being there is far more comfortable*. This is all difficult and requires a considered thought process that's unnatural and will take as long as it takes, but there is no easy quick fix. All this was the key to bringing my conscious and subconscious mind back together again. I began to learn how to confront the issues and deal with the consequences, I began to wrestle back some control.

Gradually I'd sleep on consecutive nights and then the number of sleepless nights per week reduced. Now a bad night is maybe three hours' sleep, but generally I'm sleeping every night for five to six hours and have avoided having to take any medication. I walk every night still, I think, for the pleasure of reflective, quiet me-time, in a beautiful place, rather than out of necessity. My nightly late security patrol around the village is fairly well-known now, I'm no longer the creepy dark dog less silhouette lurking in the shadows.

With the battle at home now improving, we've pushed at one or two days away, and any day that I'm fully engaged because I've had enough sleep, even with as little as three hours, is a tick in the success box, a little hard-fought victory. This progress has been delayed with the 2020 lockdown as a result of the coronavirus pandemic, but I know I can improve.

My recovery has been, well I was going to say slow, but that isn't right, there is no slow or fast. Truth is it will take as long as it takes and no matter how much you wish for it, there isn't anything you can do to speed it up and mine will likely never be totally complete. This simple fact, no matter how many times well-meaning people say it to you, can only be learnt with bumps and scrapes along the way. You fight for a period, get hurt, learn, dust yourself off and carry on. It is relentless, constant, day in day out, way longer than you may hope and well after everyone else's interest has rightly waned, but just having people there helps.

Being told that things could have been very much worse, while that is correct, doesn't really help, you are where you are and you always want more. So, have I recovered? Well yes and no, the yes is bigger than the no. I have little physical and mental deficits that remain and are likely to be constant reminders of that time for the rest of my life. Now a little over four years later there still hasn't been a day I'm not reminded of that time, a bit like a small stone in my shoe that I can't get rid of. I have images and thoughts that pop up in my head from time to time that will never dim, they just don't bother me quite as much anymore, they don't fully control me. And just a very small handful of the memories I have, out of the hundreds I've acquired, not enough to made it all worthwhile, I don't want to forget, they were wonderful.

Afterword

Peter was pre-alerted to me on the assessment unit as a patient with acute confusion and query sepsis. I was preparing Peter's bed space and monitoring equipment when he was brought up from the Emergency Department, clearly terrified and unwell. He was accompanied by his wife, Trish, who was trying very hard to keep calm and be by her husband's side. Peter was showing many of the red flags symptoms for sepsis and had received treatment on admission to the Emergency Department. I was very concerned about Peter, I spoke with the nurse-in-charge and my colleagues; as a team of doctors, nurses and healthcare assistants, we escalated and referred Peter straight away to Critical Care. He received the treatment he needed, following the Sepsis Six protocol, and I spoke to his wife to explain what we were doing, and he was transferred to Critical Care.

As nurses, we see many, many patients and some you remember, some you forget with good wishes. Some you think you know what will happen to them and then they surprise you. Peter will always be that patient for me, that person where I could see that his life was in the balance, and it would just take one small thing to tip it either way. It has been an absolute privilege to know Peter the patient, but more importantly, Peter the person.

Natasha Wilson
NGH Practice Development Nurse, Medicine and Urgent Care

I had the fortunate experience to meet Peter at a Sepsis Event that I had asked him if would attend. Prior to that I had seen pictures and videos of Peter telling of his experiences. Meeting Peter was so inspiring, not only had he fought and won the battle with this deadly disease, he was humble and grateful for the care that he had received. He also wanted to share his experiences so that other individuals who happen to experience sepsis where not muddling through the darkness.

Personally, I feel Peter is a true expert on Sepsis, he has lived it. I have learnt so much from Peter, with a critical care background the focus has always been to save the patients, early identification etc. Peter made me realise that there is a whole series of events that follow, once the patient is discharged from critical care and essentially hospital. I could not stop reading these pages once I picked them up, I feel that I am certainly a better practitioner, nurse as a result of meeting Peter and certainly a better person.

Jessica O'Sullivan
NGH Sepsis Nurse.

Acknowledgements

My wife Trish and our children, George and Kate. My brother David and his partner Hazel, who all spent so much time with me in hospital and have been so supportive and understanding during my recovery. My other brother Paul and his wife Terri who live in South Africa who, as always, I know were with me so much in spirit. Together with all my amazing extended family.

All those nurses and others who are initialled, mentioned or that I encountered, who I've been unable to contact, and I will always think of so fondly. Particular thanks to those that played their part in this story that I'm unfortunately unaware of, so was not able to thank at the time, at least you escaped the hug. Everyone else at Northampton General Hospital (NGH).

Augustus Lusack, NGH Head of Pathology, who very kindly gave up some of his time to meet with me. He was also sufficiently motivated during the 2020 coronavirus pandemic to write the foreword for me.

Dr Jonathan Hardwick, NGH ICU Consultant, Sepsis Lead: The main man. What can I say? All this in the end came down to him being able to successfully bring me through that eight seconds.

Emma Madden, NGH ICU Follow-up nurse, whose skill, experience and support at the follow-up meetings was so reassuring, also for the fabulous work she has done at Northampton ICU Steps.

Jessica O'Sulivan, NGH Sepsis Nurse. Who I met during my recovery at Sepsis Wellbeing meetings and events. She also was the first clinician to look over an early draft of this to correct things where needed. Jess was also very encouraging to get me to finally do something with this, along with Natasha.

Natasha Wilson: NGH Practice Development Nurse. Formally of Benham Assessment Unit who looked after me when I was first admitted, and I've subsequently met during my recovery.

My special village in general, and the other five Tuesday night drinkers in particular, Nigel Bould, Mark Henderson, John Quilter, Gary Wells and Duane Winter.

All those that I've shared experiences with at the Northampton ICU Steps and the Sepsis Wellbeing Group.

Grosvenor House Publishing, who so professionally guided me through the process of completing this process.

Person unknown, ref EM968 from Scribendi. The first person to read the first draft of this. Having spent a long time blowing hot and cold over whether I should do anything with this story, having got almost all I needed to out of just writing it down. I eventually mailed it to the only company I could find offering to do a manuscript critique without a proofreading and asked them to be as harsh as they liked. They were very encouraging offered good constructive advice to a first-time total novice. This gave me the confidence to have it checked for clinical errors by Jess, Tash and Gus, who I'd had the great pleasure of meeting during my recovery. Then the Tuesdayboys pub group who were guinea pigs in reading an early draft of this, just to see if I was comfortable doing it.

The interview Trish and I gave for the NGH in house magazine, was videoed and an edited version was available to watch from the NGH website, their facebook page or via the following YouTube link:

https://www.youtube.com/watch?v=Vsy5tCHULPY

Lightning Source UK Ltd.
Milton Keynes UK
UKHW010638210121
377450UK00002B/338

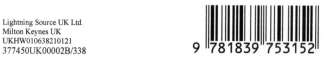

9 781839 753152